Lecture Notes
Diseases of the Ear, Nose and Throat

Peter Bull
Senior Consultant Otolaryngologist
Royal Hallamshire Hospital
Sheffield Children's Hospital
Sheffield, UK

Honorary Senior Clinical Lecturer
Department of Otolaryngology
University of Sheffield
Sheffield, UK

Ray Clarke
Consultant Otolaryngologist
Royal Liverpool Children's Hospital
Alder Hey
Liverpool, UK

Lecturer in Otolaryngology
University of Liverpool
Liverpool, UK

Tenth Edition

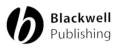

Blackwell
Publishing

© 2007 Peter Bull and Ray Clarke
Published by Blackwell Publishing

Blackwell Publishing, Inc., 350 Main Street, Malden, MA 02148-5020, USA
Blackwell Publishing Ltd, 9600 Garsington Road, Oxford OX4 2DQ, UK
Blackwell Publishing Asia Pty Ltd, 550 Swanston Street, Carlton, Victoria 3053, Australia

First published 1961   Fourth edition 1976   Seventh edition 1991   Tenth edition 2007
Second edition 1968   Fifth edition 1980   Eighth edition 1996
Third edition 1972   Sixth edition 1985   Ninth edition 2002

3   2008

Library of Congress Cataloging-in-Publication Data

Bull, P. D.
  Lecture notes. Diseases of the ear, nose and throat. — 10th ed. / Peter Bull, Ray Clarke.
    p. ; cm.
  Rev. ed. of: Lecture notes on diseases of the ear, nose, and throat. 9th ed. / P. D. Bull.
  Includes index.
  ISBN-13: 978-1-4051-4508-4 (alk. paper)
  1. Otolaryngology. I. Clarke, Ray (Raymond) II. Bull, P. D. Lecture notes on diseases
of the ear, nose, and throat. III. Title. IV. Title: Diseases of the ear, nose and throat.
  [DNLM: 1. Otorhinolaryngologic Diseases. WV 140 B935L 2007]
  RF46.B954 2007
  617.5′1—dc22

                                                                              2006100348

  ISBN: 978-1-4051-4508-4

A catalogue record for this title is available from the British Library

Set in 8/12 Stone Serif by Charon Tec Ltd (A Macmillan Company), Chennai, India
www.charontec.com
Printed and bound in Singapore by Markono Print Media Pte Ltd

Commissioning Editor: Vicki Noyes
Editorial Assistant: Robin Harries
Development Editor: Karen Moore
Production Controller: Debbie Wyer

For further information on Blackwell Publishing, visit our website:
http://www.blackwellpublishing.com

The publisher's policy is to use permanent paper from mills that operate a sustainable
forestry policy, and which has been manufactured from pulp processed using acid-free
and elementary chlorine-free practices. Furthermore, the publisher ensures that the
text paper and cover board used have met acceptable environmental accreditation
standards.

Lecture Notes
Diseases of the Ear, Nose and Throat

Contents

Contents

Preface to the tenth edition

This compact little book enjoys a niche in the affections of current and former medical students – including myself – for its clarity and focus on the core clinical principles of otolaryngology. Mr Peter Bull was sole author of the last four editions of *Lecture Notes on Diseases of the Ear, Nose and Throat*. When he asked me to help him put together this tenth edition, I was conscious of my role as custodian of an important tradition in the specialty. I have tried to retain the 'readability' which so characterised previous editions. Nevertheless, substantial revisions were needed to reflect changes not only in ENT but also in the needs and learning methods of the modern undergraduate medical student.

There are new chapters and sections on head and neck cancer, benign neck disease, obstructive sleep apnoea, adenotonsillar disease, otitis media and the management of deafness. Some 40 new figures have been added. Many chapters have been shortened to maintain the brevity that is so important in a modern curriculum. As a thorough knowledge of anatomy and physiology can no longer be assumed in students at the time they study ENT, there is enough applied basic science to make the clinical material understandable. To emphasise integration between basic science and clinical work, this material lies mainly at the start of relevant chapters. Each chapter now ends with one or more 'nuggets of wisdom' (clinical practice points), and in response to student demand I have added a self-assessment section consisting of multiple choice questions. This is intended as a learning aid rather than a practice examination.

Mr Peter Bull, my teacher and mentor, retires from clinical and teaching practice this year. I hope my contribution to this tenth edition will be seen as a tribute to his skills as a first-rate teacher and surgeon who had an immensely positive influence on the education of several generations of young – and not so young – doctors. No doubt this book will further evolve. I am open to feedback and ask readers to email me with any suggestions so that they may be incorporated in future editions: Raymond.Clarke@rlc.nhs.uk.

Ray Clarke
Liverpool

Chapter 1

The ear: some applied basic science

The pinna

The external ear or pinna is composed of cartilage with closely adherent peri-chondrium and skin. It is developed from six tubercles of the first branchial arch. Fistulae and accessory auricles result from failure of fusion of these tubercles.

The external auditory meatus or ear canal

The external auditory meatus is about 25 mm in length, has a skeleton of cartilage in its outer third (where it contains hairs and ceruminous or 'wax-producing' glands) and has bone in its inner two-thirds. The skin of the inner part is exceedingly thin, adherent and sensitive. Wax, debris or foreign bodies may lodge in an antero-inferior recess at the medial end of the meatus.

The tympanic membrane or eardrum (Fig. 1.1)

The tympanic membrane is composed of three layers from out to in – skin, fibrous tissue and mucosa. The normal appearance of the membrane is pearly and opaque. When light reflects off the drum it forms a characteristic triangular 'light reflex' due to its concave shape. If you see this 'light reflex', that is good evidence that the drum is normal.

The tympanic cavity or middle ear

Medial to the eardrum, the tympanic cavity is an air-containing space 15 mm high and 15 mm antero-posteriorly, although only 2 mm deep in parts. The middle ear contains the small middle-ear bones the malleus, incus and stapes ('hammer', 'anvil' and 'stirrup' (Figs 1.2 and 1.3). Its medial wall is crowded with structures

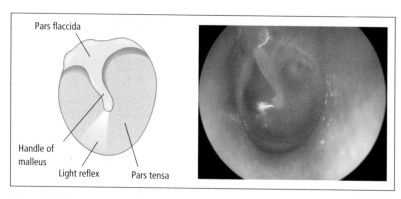

Figure 1.1 The normal tympanic membrane (left). The shape of the incus is visible through the drum at 2 o'clock (courtesy of MPJ Yardley). The 'pars flaccida' in the upper part of the drum is thinner than the 'pars tensa' as the middle fibrous layer is defective.

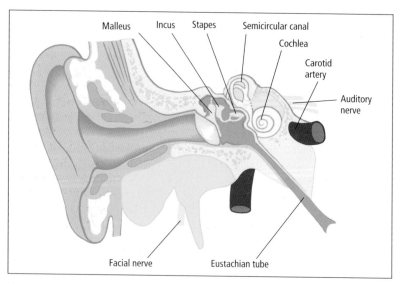

Figure 1.2 Diagram to show the relationship between the external, middle and inner ears.

closely related to one another: the facial nerve, the round and oval windows, the lateral semicircular canal and basal turn of the cochlea.

The Eustachian tube

The Eustachian tube connects the middle-ear cleft with the nasopharynx at the back of the nasal cavity. The tube permits aeration of the middle ear and if it is

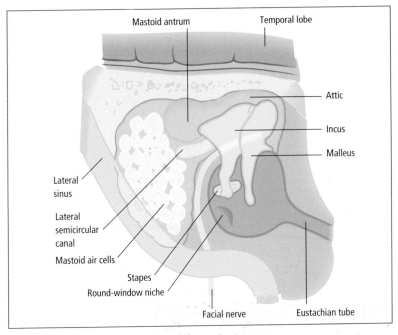

Figure 1.3 Diagram to show the anatomy of the middle ear and mastoid air cells.

obstructed fluid may accumulate in the middle ear causing deafness. The tube is shorter, wider and more horizontal in the infant than in the adult. Secretions or food may enter the tympanic cavity more easily in the supine position particularly during feeding in babies. The tube is normally closed and opens on swallowing because of movement of the muscles of the palate. This movement is impaired in cleft palate children who often develop accumulation of middle-ear fluid.

The inner ear

The inner ear is made up of the cochlea, responsible for hearing and the semicircular canals which house the 'balance organs'. The delicate neuroepithelium is well protected in the dense petrous part of the temporal bone (Figs 1.4 and 1.5).

The facial nerve

The facial nerve is the motor nerve to the muscles of facial expression. Intimately associated with the ear, it is embedded in the temporal bone and passes through

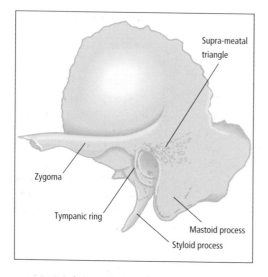

Supra-meatal triangle

Zygoma

Tympanic ring

Mastoid process

Styloid process

Figure 1.4 The left temporal bone.

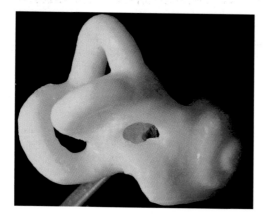

Figure 1.5 A preparation showing the bony inner ear of semicircular canals and cochlea (preparation by Mr S. Ell).

the middle ear but exits the skull at the stylomastoid foramen just in front of the mastoid process. In infants, the mastoid process is undeveloped and the nerve is very superficial.

The mastoid cells

The mastoid cells form a honeycomb within the temporal bone, acting as a reservoir of air to limit pressure changes within the middle ear. The extent of pneumatization is very variable and is usually reduced in chronic middle-ear disease when the mastoid is often said to be 'sclerotic'.

The mechanism of hearing

Sound causes the eardrum to vibrate. This energy is transmitted via the ossicles to the oval window which is in contact with the stapes. A 'travelling wave' is set up in the fluids of the inner ear. Specialized neuroepithelial cells ('hair cells') in the cochlea or inner ear convert this energy to nerve impulses which then travel along the auditory pathway to the cortex where they are recognized as sound. Diseases which interfere with transmission of sound across the 'outer' and 'middle' ear cause 'conductive' deafness, and diseases in the 'inner ear' which interfere with the conversion of this energy to nerve impulses or with the transmission of these nerve impulses cause sensorineural or 'nerve' deafness.

Clinical practice points

- The facial nerve is intimately related to the middle and inner ears. Always check the ear carefully in a patient with facial palsy.
- The middle ear amplifies sound. The inner ear is essential for hearing. Middle-ear disease may cause some degree of deafness but if the inner ear is not functioning the patient will be completely deaf in that ear.

5

Chapter 2

Clinical examination of the ear

The examination of the ear includes close inspection of the pinna, the external auditory canal and the eardrum. Scars from any previous surgery may be inconspicuous and easily missed. Make sure you gently tilt the pinna forward and look behind the ear for a post-aural scar.

The ear is most conveniently examined with an auriscope or 'otoscope' (Fig. 2.1). Modern auriscopes have distal illumination via a fibre-optic cone giving a bright,

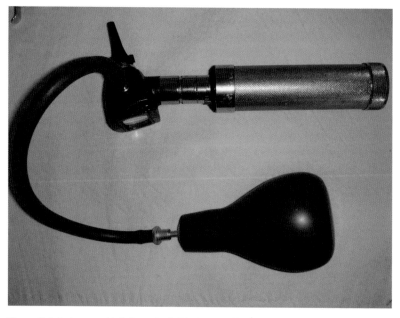

Figure 2.1 Auriscope with halogen bulb lighting via a fibre-optic cone. Note the bulb which is for pneumatic otoscopy.

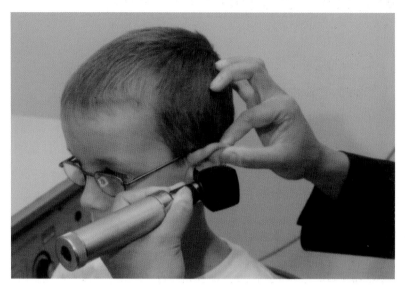

Figure 2.2 The best method for holding the auriscope.

even light. Because interpretation of the appearance depends to a large extent on colour, it is essential that the battery should be in good condition to give a white light.

A common error in examination of the ear is to use too small a speculum; it is a mistake to think this is gentler – use the largest speculum that can be easily inserted (Fig. 2.2). A good otoscope is expensive but a worthwhile investment. There may be an attachment which permits insufflation of air into the ear canal so that the mobility of the drum can be assessed – pneumatic otoscopy. Important points in the examination of the ear are listed in Box 2.1.

Clinical practice points

- Make sure you use the biggest speculum that fits in the ear canal.
- Be gentle; otoscopy in a non-inflamed ear should be completely painless.

Box 2.1   Examination of the ear

1 Look for any scars.

2 Examine the pinna and outer meatus in a good light – you can use the auriscope for this.

3 Remove any wax or debris by syringing, or by instruments if you are practised in this.

4 Pull the pinna gently backwards and upwards (downwards and backwards in infants) to straighten out the meatus.

5 Insert the auriscope *gently* into the meatus and see where you are going by looking *through* the instrument. If you cannot get a good view, either the speculum is the wrong size or the angulation is wrong.

6 Inspect the external canal.

7 Inspect all parts of the tympanic membrane by varying the angle of the speculum.

8 Do not be satisfied until you have seen the membrane completely.

9 The normal appearance of the membrane varies and can only be learnt by practice. Such practice will lead to the recognition of subtle abnormalities as well as the more obvious ones.

Chapter 3

Testing the hearing

Audiograms can be wrong.
There are three stages to testing the hearing and all are important.
1 Clinical assessment of the degree of deafness.
2 Tuning fork tests.
3 Audiometry.

Clinical assessment of the degree of deafness

By talking to the patient, the examiner quickly appreciates how well a patient can hear and this assessment continues throughout the interview. Voice and whisper tests are approximations but with practice can be a good guide to the level of hearing. Make a more formal assessment by asking the patient to repeat words spoken by the examiner at different intensities and distances in each ear in turn. Sit beside the patient and use one hand to occlude the ear canal gently in the non-test ear (masking). This will mean that the examiners voice is approximately 1 metre from the test ear (Fig. 3.1). Record the result as, for example, whispered voice (WV) at 1 metre in a patient with slight deafness, or conversational voice (CV) at 1 metre in a deafer individual.

If profound unilateral deafness is suspected, the good ear should be more thoroughly masked with a specially designed noise box (Barany noise box) and the deaf ear tested by shouting into it.

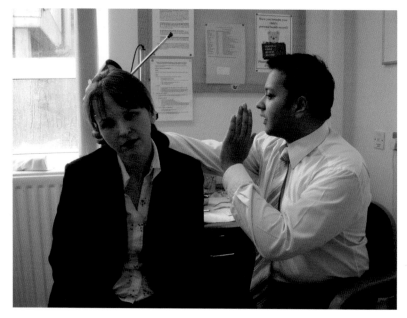

Figure 3.1 Testing the hearing by voice. The tester should shield his/her mouth from the patient to prevent lipreading.

Tuning fork tests

Before considering tuning fork tests it is necessary to have a basic concept of classification of deafness. Almost every form of deafness (and there are many) may be classified under one of these headings:
- Conductive deafness.
- Sensorineural deafness.
- Mixed conductive and sensorineural deafness.

Conductive deafness (Fig. 3.2)

Conductive deafness results from failure of transmission of sound waves across the outer or middle ear, preventing sound energy from reaching the cochlear fluids. It may be improved by surgery and so it is important to recognize.

Sensorineural deafness (Fig. 3.2)

Sensorineural deafness results from defective function of the cochlea or of the auditory nerve. This prevents neural impulses from being transmitted to the auditory cortex of the brain.

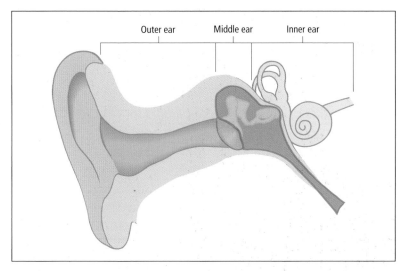

Outer ear   Middle ear   Inner ear

Figure 3.2 Sensorineural deafness is caused by an abnormality of the cochlea or the auditory nerve (inner ear). Conductive deafness is caused by abnormality of the outer or middle ear.

Mixed deafness

Mixed deafness is the term used to describe a combination of conductive and sensorineural deafness in the same ear.

Rinne's test

This test compares the relative effectiveness of sound transmission through the middle ear by air conduction (AC), and bypassing the middle ear by bone conduction (BC). It is usually performed as follows: a tuning fork of 512 Hz (cycles per second) is struck and held close to the patient's ear (AC); the base is then placed firmly on the mastoid process behind the ear (BC) and the patient is asked to state whether it is heard better by BC or AC (Fig. 3.3).

Interpretation of Rinne's test

If AC > BC (called Rinne positive) the middle and outer ears are functioning normally.

If BC > AC (called Rinne negative) there is defective function of the outer or middle ear (conductive deafness).

Rinne's test tells you little or nothing about the cochlea. It is a test of middle-ear function.

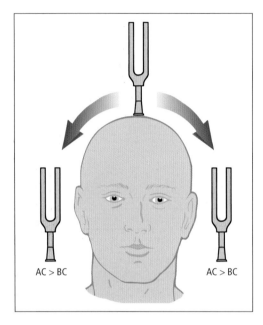

AC > BC   AC > BC

Figure 3.3 Tuning fork tests showing a positive Rinne in each ear and the Weber test referred equally to each ear, indicating symmetrical hearing in both ears with normal middle-ear function.

Weber's test

This test is useful in determining the type of deafness and in deciding which ear has the better-functioning cochlea. The base of a vibrating tuning fork is held on the middle of the skull and the patient is asked whether the sound is heard centrally or is referred to one or other ear.

In conductive deafness the sound is heard in the deafer ear.

In sensorineural deafness the sound is heard in the better-hearing ear (Figs 3.3–3.5).

Audiometry

Pure tone audiometry

Pure tone audiometry provides a measurement of hearing levels by AC and BC and depends on the cooperation of the subject. The test should be carried out in a sound-proofed room. The audiometer is an instrument that generates pure tone signals ranging from 125 to 12,000 Hz (12 kHz) at variable intensities. The signal is fed to the patient through earphones (for AC) or a small vibrator applied to the mastoid process (for BC). Signals of increasing intensity at each

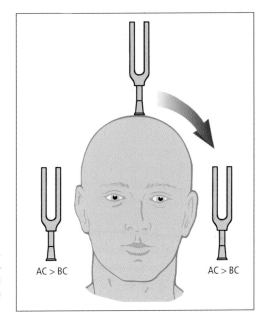

Figure 3.4 Sensorineural deafness in the right ear. The Rinne test is positive on both sides and the Weber test is referred to the left ear.

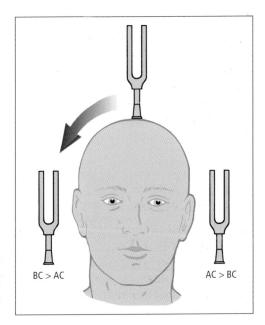

Figure 3.5 Conductive deafness in the right ear. The Rinne test is negative on the right, positive on the left, and the Weber test is referred to the right ear.

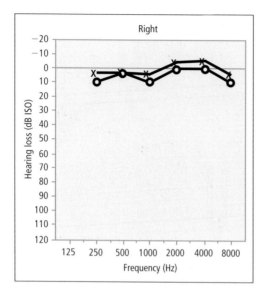

Figure 3.6 A normal pure tone audiogram. o–o–o, right ear; x–x–x, left ear.

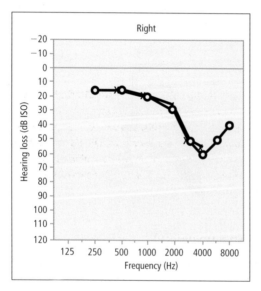

Figure 3.7 A pure tone audiogram showing sensorineural deafness maximal at 4 kHz typical of noise-induced deafness.

frequency are fed to the patient, who indicates when the test tone can be heard. The threshold of hearing at each frequency is charted in the form of an audiogram (Figs 3.6–3.8), with hearing loss expressed in decibels (dB). Decibels are logarithmic units of relative intensity of sound energy. When testing hearing

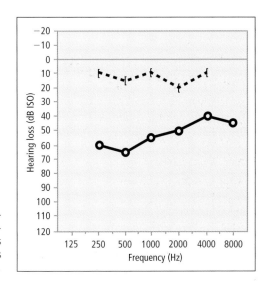

Figure 3.8 A pure tone audio-gram showing conductive deafness. The BC (dashed line) is normal but the AC (solid line) is impaired. A case of otosclerosis.

by BC, it is essential to mask the opposite ear with narrow-band noise to avoid cross-transmission of the signal to that ear.

Speech audiometry

Speech audiometry measures the ability of each ear to discriminate the spoken word at different intensities. A recorded word list is supplied to the patient through the audiometer at increasing loudness levels, and the score is plotted on a graph. In some disorders, the intelligibility of speech may fall above a certain intensity level. This usually implies the presence of *loudness recruitment*. Above a critical threshold, sounds are suddenly perceived as having become excessively loud. This is indicative of cochlear disorder.

Impedance audiometry (tympanometery)

Impedance audiometry measures not hearing but the compliance or mobility of the middle-ear structures. A pure tone signal of known intensity is fed into the external auditory canal via an ear probe and a microphone in the probe measures reflected sound levels. Thus, the sound admitted to the ear can be measured. Most sound is absorbed when the compliance is maximal and by altering the pressure in the external canal, a measure can be made of the compliance at different pressures. Impedance testing is widely used as a screening method for otitis media with effusion (OME) in children. If there is fluid in the middle ear, the compliance curve is flattened.

Electric response audiometry

Electric response audiometry is a collective term for investigations whereby nerve activity in the form of action potentials (APs) at various points within the long and complex auditory pathway can be recorded. The AP is evoked by a sound stimulus applied to the ear and the resulting AP is collected in a computer store. Although each AP is tiny, it occurs at the same time interval after the stimulus (usually a click of *very* short duration) and so a train of stimuli will produce an easily detectable response. By making the computer look at different time windows, responses at various sites in the auditory pathway can be investigated.

Electric response audiometry has the unique advantage of being an objective measure of hearing requiring no cooperation from the subject. It is of value in assessing hearing thresholds in babies and small children and in cases of dispute such as litigation for industrial deafness.

Otoacoustic emissions

When the ear is subjected to a sound wave it is stimulated to produce itself an emission of sound generated within the cochlea. This can be detected and recorded and has been used as a screening test of hearing in newborn babies. It is now in routine clinical use in testing those babies who are particularly at risk of hearing problems, such as premature or hypoxic neonates, and is used in screening babies for deafness.

Clinical practice point

• Otoacoustic emissions (OAEs) are a quick and non-invasive way to test for hearing in newborn babies.

Chapter 4

Deafness

Attention has already been drawn to the two major categories of deafness – conductive and sensorineural. The distinction is easily made by tuning fork tests, which should never be omitted.

Causes

There is no strict order in the list featured in Table 4.1, because the frequency with which various causes of deafness occur varies from one community to another and from one age group to another. Nevertheless, some indication is given by division into 'more common' and 'less common' groups. Some deterioration in hearing acuity is a normal feature of ageing, sometimes associated with tinnitus or 'noises in the ear'. Always try to make a diagnosis of the cause of deafness and start by deciding whether it is conductive or sensorineural.

The deaf child

The commonest cause of deafness in children is fluid in the middle ear due to otitis media. This causes a temporary conductive deafness. Sensorineural loss is rare (one in a thousand newborns) but nearly always permanent. Early diagnosis of deafness in babies is essential to avoid irretrievable delay in language development. The mother's assessment is important and should always be taken seriously. Some babies are 'at risk' of deafness and are tested as soon after birth as possible. They include those with:
1 prematurity and low birth-weight;
2 perinatal hypoxia;

3 Rhesus disease;

4 family history of hereditary deafness;

5 intrauterine exposure to viruses such as rubella, cytomegalovirus and HIV.

The testing of babies suspected or at risk of being deaf is very specialized.

Sudden sensorineural deafness

Sudden deafness may be unilateral or bilateral and most cases are regarded as being viral or vascular. Sudden sensorineural deafness is an emergency and should be treated seriously. Bilateral profound deafness, especially if sudden, is a devastating event. Arrange admission to hospital as delay may mean permanent deafness.

Investigation may show no cause and treatment is usually with low-molecular-weight dextran, steroids and inhaled carbon dioxide in an attempt to improve blood flow to the inner ear, although there is no good evidence that these strategies are effective.

Table 4.1 Causes of deafness

Conductive	Sensorineural
More common	
Wax	Presbycusis (deafness of old age)
Acute otitis media	Noise-induced (prolonged exposure to high noise level, industrial deafness, disco music)
Barotrauma	Congenital (maternal rubella, cytomegalovirus,
Otosclerosis	toxoplasmosis, hereditary deafness, anoxia, jaundice, congenital syphilis)
Injury of the tympanic membrane	Drug-induced (aminoglycoside antibiotics, aspirin, quinine, some diuretics, some beta blockers)
	Menière's disease
	Late otosclerosis
	Infections (Chronic otitis media, mumps, herpes zoster, meningitis, syphilis)
Less common	
Traumatic ossicular dislocation	Vestibular Schwannoma
Congenital atresia of the external canal	Head injury
Agenesis of the middle ear	CNS disease (multiple sclerosis, metastases)
Tumours of the middle ear	Metabolic (diabetes, hypothyroidism, Paget's disease of bone)
	Unknown aetiology

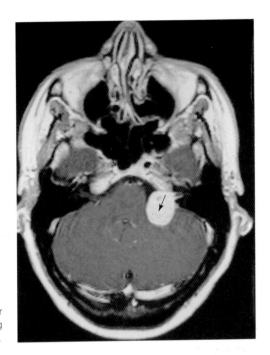

Figure 4.1 An MR scan after gadolinium contrast showing an acoustic neuroma (arrowed).

Vestibular Schwannoma (acoustic neuroma)

Vestibular Schwannoma is a benign nerve tumour in the internal auditory meatus or cerebello-pontine (CP) angle at the base of the skull. It is usually unilateral, except in the very rare familial neurofibromatosis type 2 (NF2), when it may be bilateral. In its early stages, it causes progressive hearing loss and imbalance. As it enlarges, it may encroach on the trigeminal nerve in the CP angle, causing loss of corneal sensation. In its advanced stage, there is raised intracranial pressure and brain stem displacement. Early diagnosis reduces the morbidity and mortality. Unilateral sensorineural deafness should always be investigated to exclude a neuroma. Audiometry will confirm the hearing loss. MR scanning will identify even small tumours (Fig. 4.1).

Hearing aids

Hearing aids work on the principle of amplifying sound. In the typical 'behind the ear' aid a small microphone picks up sound which is then amplified electronically and fed into the ear canal by an earpiece or mould customized to fit the patient's ear canal. The amplifier is housed behind the ear. More sophisticated

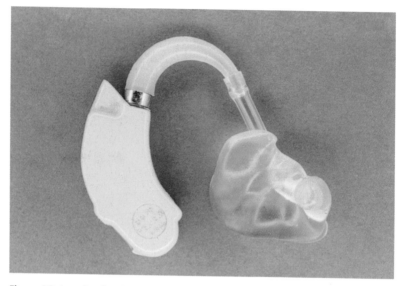

Figure 4.2 A modern hearing aid.

(and expensive) are the 'all-in-the-ear' aids, where the electronics are built into a mould made to fit the patient's ear. Some patients prefer these as they are inconspicuous. They give good directional hearing and, because they are individually built, the output can be matched to the patient's deafness. Modern hearing aids are digital, allowing more refinement in the sound processing and more control of the aid. Whatever the capacity of the aid for amplification there are problems with clarity for many deaf patients. In cochlear forms of sensorineural deafness, loudness recruitment is often marked. This results in an intolerance of noise above a certain threshold, making amplification very difficult. Many modern hearing aids are fitted with a loop inductance system to make the use of telephones easier (Fig. 4.2).

Bone-anchored hearing aids

Some patients are unable to use a conventional hearing aid because of the shape of the ear canal or due to chronic infection. They may be suitable for a bone-anchored hearing aid (BAHA). A titanium screw is threaded into the temporal bone and allowed to fuse to the bone (osseo-integration). This allows the attachment of a special hearing aid that transmits sound directly by bone conduction to the cochlea (Fig. 4.3).

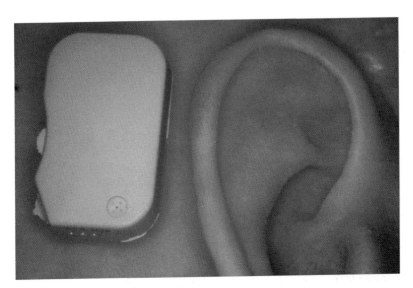

Figure 4.3 A bone-anchored hearing aid.

Cochlear implants

These rely on the implantation of electrodes into the cochlea to stimulate the auditory nerve. The apparatus consists of a microphone, an electronic sound processor and an electrode implanted into the cochlea. Cochlear implantation is only appropriate for bilateral profound deafness. Results can be spectacular, with some patients able to converse easily. Most patients obtain a significant improvement in their ability to communicate (Fig. 4.4).

Lip-reading

Instruction in lip-reading is much more effective while usable hearing persists and should always be offered to those at risk of total or profound deafness.

Sign language

Many deaf children and adults learn to communicate very effectively by sign language.

Electronic aids for the deaf

Amplifying telephones, flashing alarms and vibrating alert devices are available to the deaf.

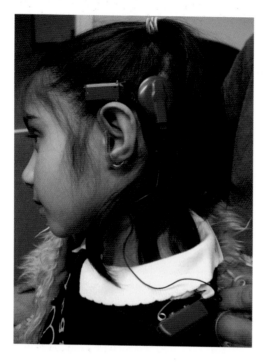

Figure 4.4 A child with cochlear implant. Picture courtesy Mr. CH Raine FRCS.

Clinical practice points

- Early identification of childhood deafness makes for a greatly improved outcome. Take the mother's concerns seriously.
- Unilateral sensorineural deafness should be investigated to exclude a neuroma.

Chapter 5

Conditions of the pinna

Congenital

Protruding ears

Sometimes unkindly known as 'bat ears', the terms protruding or prominent should be used. The underlying deformity is the absence of the ante-helical fold in the auricular cartilage (Figs 5.1 and 5.2). Affected children are often teased

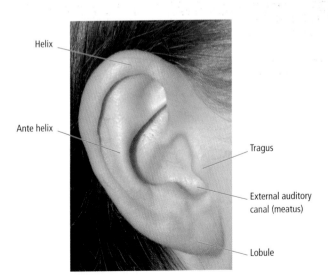

Helix

Ante helix

Tragus

External auditory
canal (meatus)

Lobule

Figure 5.1 Parts of the pinna.

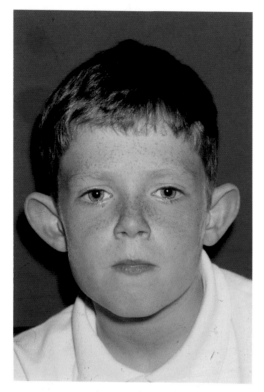

Figure 5.2 A child with protruding ears.

mercilessly and surgical correction can be carried out after the age of four. The operation consists of exposing the lateral aspect of the cartilage from behind the pinna and scoring it to produce a rounded fold.

Accessory auricles

Accessory auricles are small tags, often containing cartilage, on a line between the angle of the mouth and the tragus (Fig. 5.3). They may be multiple.

Pre-auricular sinus

Pre-auricular sinus is a small blind pit that occurs most commonly anterior to the root of the helix; it is sometimes bilateral and may be familial. If they become recurrently infected they are best excised (Fig. 5.4).

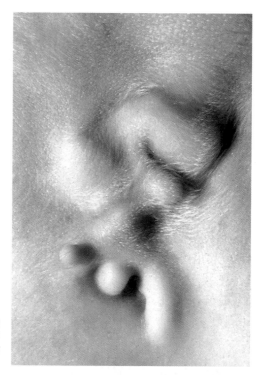

Figure 5.3 Right ear showing congenital meatal atresia, an accessory auricle and deformity of the pinna.

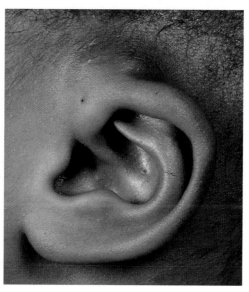

Figure 5.4 Pre-auricular sinus.

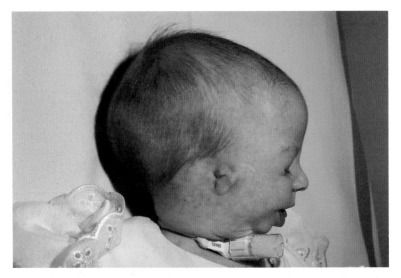

Figure 5.5 A child with Treacher Collins syndrome.

Microtia

Microtia, or failure of development of the pinna, may be associated with atresia of the ear canal (Fig. 5.3). Absence or severe malformation of the external ear, as in Treacher Collins syndrome (Fig. 5.5), may be remedied by the fitting of prosthetic ears attached by bone-anchored titanium screws (see BAHA, Chapter 4, pages 20–21). A bone-anchored hearing aid can be fitted at the same time, although it is often fitted at a much earlier age than prosthetic ears in order to allow speech development.

Trauma

Subperichondrial haematoma of the pinna usually occurs as a result of a shearing blow (Fig. 5.6). The pinna is ballooned and the outline of the cartilage is lost. As the blood supply of the cartilage is from the perichondrium, an untreated haematoma will cause severe deformity – a cauliflower ear. Treatment consists of evacuation of the clot and the reapposition of cartilage and perichondrium by pressure dressings or vacuum drain.

Avulsion

Very rarely, the pinna can be avulsed. If the avulsed ear is preserved, and quickly reattached surgically, survival of the tissues may be possible.

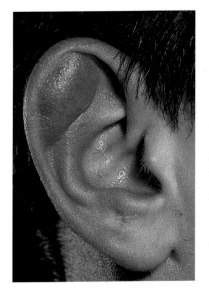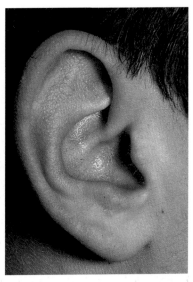

Figure 5.6 Auricular haematoma before and after drainage.

Inflammation

Acute dermatitis

Extension of meatal infection in otitis externa can cause acute dermatitis of the pinna, as can a sensitivity reaction to topically applied antibiotics, especially chloramphenicol or neomycin (Fig. 5.7).

Treatment

1 The ear canal should be adequately cleaned (q.v.).
2 If there is any suspicion of a sensitivity reaction, topical treatment with antibiotics should be withdrawn.
3 The ear may be treated by a glycerine and ichthammol wick, or an emollient ointment.
4 Steroid ointment may be applied *sparingly*.
5 Severe cases may require admission to hospital.

Perichondritis

Perichondritis may follow injury to the cartilage, mastoid surgery or ear piercing, particularly with the modern trend for multiple perforations that go

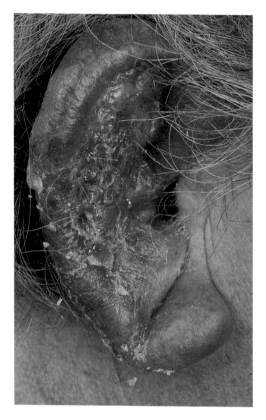

Figure 5.7 Severe otitis externa and perichondritis of the pinna.

through the cartilage. Treatment must be vigorous, with parenteral antibiotics and incision if necessary. If it is due to piercing the stud should be removed.

Chondrodermatitis chronicis helicis

Chondrodermatitis chronicis helicis occurs in the elderly as a painful ulcerated lesion on the rim of the helix. It resembles a neoplasm and should be removed for histology.

Tumours

Squamous cell and basal cell carcinomas

These skin tumours occur usually on the upper edge of the pinna. They are related to exposure to sunlight and when small are easily treated by local excision.

Large tumours of the pinna or outer meatus will require more radical treatment, often with skin flap repair.

Clinical practice point

• If otitis externa gets worse on topical treatment, it is probably due to drug sensitivity. Stop the treatment.

Chapter 6

Conditions of the external auditory meatus

Congenital

'*Atresia*' (Greek: a, negative; tretos, bored through) is a failure of development; in the case of the ear there may be a shallow blind pit or no opening at all. The pinna may be small (*microtia*) or missing (*anotia*) and the middle or inner ear may be poorly developed or even absent (Fig. 5.3).

Atresia of the ear is a feature of many syndromes in childhood and as congenital anomalies are often multiple, a careful assessment of the baby's general health is essential. It is particularly important to assess the hearing. If the child has hearing impairment, rehabilitation in the form of hearing aids should commence immediately. Correction of the deformity of the external and middle ear can be delayed until the child is old enough to participate in the decision-making. The bone-anchored hearing aid (BAHA, see Chapter 4) and the use of titanium implants to mount a prosthesis have greatly improved the management of these children.

Foreign body

Small children often put beads, pips, paper and other objects into their own ears, but they will usually blame someone else! Adults may get a foreign body stuck in an attempt to clean the ear, e.g. with matchsticks or cotton buds. The chief danger lies in clumsy attempts to remove the foreign body. Apart from frightening the child and making any further attempts difficult this can cause abrasions to the external ear canal or even rupture of the tympanic membrane. Gentle syringing will often remove a foreign body. If you are experienced in using instruments in the ear canal you may be able to get the foreign body out with a forceps or hook. In the ENT department, an operating microscope may help to view the ear canal. Most foreign bodies are inert and there is no urgency dealing with them. An exception is the 'button battery' which needs to be removed promptly before it leaks corrosive material. Another is a live insect, such as a moth or fly, in the outer meatus. They produce dramatic 'tinnitus' and great distress. Peace is restored by the instillation of spirit or olive oil before they are syringed out.

If the child (or adult) is uncooperative, do not persevere, arrange a general anaesthetic.

Wax

Wax or cerumen produced by the ceruminous glands in the outer ear migrates laterally along the meatus. Some people produce large amounts of wax but many cases of impacted wax are due to the use of cotton wool buds in a misguided attempt to clean the ears. Ears are 'self-cleaning'!

Impacted wax may cause some deafness or irritation of the meatal skin. It is most easily removed by syringing (see Box 6.1).

Box 6.1 Ear syringing procedure

1 *History*: Has the patient had a discharging ear? If any possibility of a perforation, do not syringe.

2 *Inspection*: If wax seems very hard, always soften over a period of 1 week by using warm olive oil drops nightly. In the case of exceedingly stubborn wax, advise the patient to use sodium bicarbonate eardrops (BPC). There are 'quick-acting' ceruminolytic agents on the market. Occasionally, a patient reacts badly to these and develops otitis externa. Do not use them in patients known to suffer from recurrent infections of the ear canal.

3 *Towels*: Protect the patient well with towels and waterproofs. He will not be amused by having his clothing soaked.

4 *Lighting*: Use a good light, preferably a mirror or lamp.

5 *Solution*: Sodium bicarbonate, 4–5 g to 500 mL, or normal saline is ideal. Tap water is satisfactory.

6 *Solution temperature*: This is vital. It should be 38°C (100°F). Any departure of more than a few degrees may cause dizziness.

7 *Tools*: Metal syringes and Bacon syringes are capable of applying high pressures and the nozzle may also do damage. The preferred instrument is an electrically driven water pump with a small hand-held nozzle and a foot operated control (Fig. 6.1). It provides an elegant means of ear syringing.

8 *Direction*: Direct the stream along the roof of the auditory canal (Fig. 6.2).

9 *Inspection*: After removal of wax, inspect thoroughly to make sure none remains.

10 *Drying*: Mop excess solution from the ear. Stagnation predisposes to otitis externa.

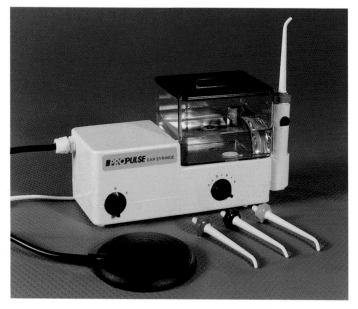

Figure 6.1 An electric pulse pump used for ear syringing.

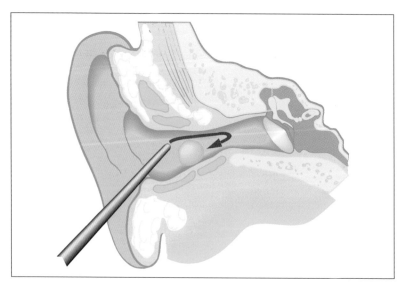

Figure 6.2 The stream of solution when syringing an ear should be directed along the roof of the external auditory canal.

Otitis externa

Otitis externa is a diffuse inflammation of the skin lining the outer ear canal. It may be bacterial or fungal (otomycosis). Irritation, desquamation, scanty discharge and a tendency to relapse are common. The treatment is simple, but success is absolutely dependent upon patience, care and meticulous attention to detail.

Causes

Some people are particularly prone to otitis externa, often because of a narrow or tortuous external canal. Most people can allow water into their ears with impunity; in others otitis externa is the inevitable result. Increased sweating and bathing in hot climates are predisposing factors. Swimming pools are a common source of otitis externa. Poking the ear with a finger or towel further traumatizes the skin and introduces new organisms. Further irritation leads to further interference with the ear, so causing more trauma. A vicious circle is set up.

Underlying skin disease such as eczema or psoriasis in the ear canal may produce very refractory otitis externa.

Ear syringing, especially if it causes trauma, may cause otitis externa.

Pathology

A mixed infection of varying organisms is typical; the most common are:
- *Staphylococcus pyogenes.*
- *Pseudomonas pyocyanea.*
- Diphtheroids.
- *Proteus vulgaris.*
- *Escherichia coli.*
- *Streptococcus faecalis.*
- *Aspergillus niger* (Fig. 6.3).
- *Candida albicans.*

Symptoms

1 Irritation (itchiness).
2 Discharge (scanty).
3 Pain (usually moderate, sometimes severe, increased by jaw movement).
4 Deafness (mild).

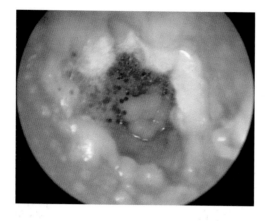

Figure 6.3 Fungal otitis externa showing the spores of *Aspergillus niger* (courtesy of MPJ Yardley).

Signs

1 Meatal tenderness, especially on movement of the pinna or compression of the tragus.
2 Moist debris, often smelly and keratotic, the removal of which reveals red desquamated skin and oedema of the meatal walls and often the tympanic membrane.

Management

Aural toilet

Scrupulous aural toilet is the key to successful treatment of otitis externa. Clean the debris and keep the ear clean and dry. No medication will be effective if the ear is full of debris and pus. Aural toilet can be done most conveniently by dry mopping. Apply a piece of fluffed-up cotton wool about the size of a postage stamp to a probe and, under direct vision, clean the ear with a gentle rotatory action. Once the cotton wool is soiled replace it (Fig. 6.4). Pay particular attention to the antero-inferior recess, which may be difficult to clean. Gentle syringing is also permissible to clear the debris.

Dressings

If the otitis externa is severe, gently insert a length of 1 cm ribbon gauze, impregnated with medication, into the meatus. Renew daily until the meatus has returned to normal. If it does not do so within 7–10 days, think again!

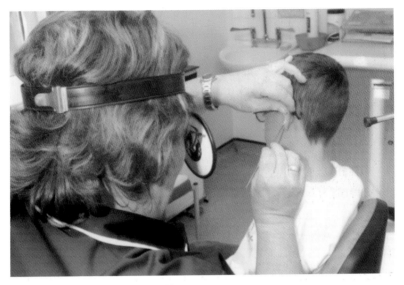

Figure 6.4 Dry mopping the ear in otitis externa.

The following medications are of value on the dressing:
1 8% aluminium acetate.
2 10% ichthammol in glycerine.
3 Ointment of gramicidin, neomycin, nystatin and triamcinolone (Tri-Adcortyl™).
4 Other medication as dictated by the result of culture.

In *fungal otitis externa* use dressings of 3% amphotericin, miconazole or nystatin.

If the otitis externa is *less severe* and there is little meatal swelling, it may respond to a combination of antibiotic and steroid eardrops. The antibiotics most commonly used are neomycin, gramicidin and framycetin but there are increasing worries about the use of aminoglycoside drops in the ear as if they reach the inner ear that can cause deafness. If there is any concern about a perforated eardrum, ciprofloxacin drops, as used in eye drops, are preferable. Remember that prolonged use may result in fungal infection or in contact dermatitis.

Prevention of recurrence

Prevention of recurrence is not always possible; the patient should be advised to keep the ears dry, especially when washing the hair or showering. A large piece

35

of cotton wool coated in Vaseline and placed in the concha is advisable, and if the patient is very keen to swim it is worthwhile investing in custom-made silicone rubber earplugs. The use of a proprietary preparation of spirit and acetic acid prophylactically after swimming is useful in reducing otitis externa. Equally important is the avoidance of scratching and poking the ears. Itching may be controlled with antihistamines given orally, especially at bedtime. If meatal stenosis predisposes to recurrent infection, meatoplasty (surgical enlargement of meatus) may be advisable.

Do not make a diagnosis of otitis externa until you have satisfied yourself that the tympanic membrane is intact. If the ear fails to settle, look again and again to make sure that you are not dealing with a case of otitis media with a discharging perforation.

Furunculosis

Furunculosis ('boil') of the external canal results from infection of a hair follicle in the lateral part of the meatus. The organism is usually *Staphylococcus*.

Symptoms

Pain

Pain is as severe as that of renal colic and the patient may need pethidine. The pain is made much worse by movement of the pinna or pressure on the tragus.

Deafness

Deafness is usually slight and due to meatal occlusion by the furuncle.

Signs

There is often no visible lesion but the introduction of an aural speculum causes intense pain. If the furuncle is larger, it will be seen as a red swelling in the outer meatus and there may be more than one furuncle present. At a more advanced stage, the furuncle will be seen to be pointing or may present as a fluctuant abscess.

Treatment

The insertion of a wick soaked in 10% ichthammol in glycerine (Glyc & Ic) or Tri-Adcortyl™ is painful at the time but provides rapid relief. Flucloxacillin should be given parenterally for 24h, followed by oral medication. Severe cases may need incision under a general anaesthetic.

Analgesics – sometimes narcotics – are essential. Recurrent cases are not common – exclude diabetes and take a nasal swab in case the patient is a *Staphylococcus* carrier.

Exostoses

Exostoses (bony overgrowths) or small osteomata of the external auditory meatus are fairly common and usually bilateral. They are much more common in those who swim a lot in cold water, although the reason is not known.

There may be two or three little tumours arising in each bony meatus. They are sessile, hard, smooth, covered with very thin skin and are often exquisitely sensitive when gently probed. Their rate of growth is extremely slow and they may give rise to no symptoms, but if wax or debris accumulates between the tympanic membrane and the exostoses, its removal may tax the patience of the most skilled manipulator. In such cases, surgical removal of the exostoses may be indicated and is carried out with the aid of the operating microscope and drill.

Malignant disease

Malignant disease of the auditory meatus is rare and usually occurs only in the elderly. If confined to the outer meatus, it behaves like skin cancer and can be treated by wide excision and skin grafting. If it spreads to invade the middle ear, facial nerve and temporomandibular joint, it is a relentless and terrible affliction. Pain becomes intractable and intolerable and there is a blood-stained discharge from the ear.

Treatment then is by radiotherapy, radical surgery or a combination of the two. Treatment is not possible in some cases, and the outlook is poor in the extreme.

Clinical practice points

- Earwax is normal and ears are self-cleaning. They do not need cotton buds, hair clips or pencils.
- Do not make a diagnosis of otitis externa until you have satisfied yourself that the tympanic membrane is intact. If the ear fails to settle, look again and again to make sure that you are not dealing with a case of otitis media with a discharging perforation.
- Meticulous aural toilet is the key to treating otitis externa.

Chapter 7

Injury of the tympanic membrane

The tympanic membrane is well protected. Traumatic damage when it does occur may be direct or indirect.

Direct trauma can be caused by poking in the ear with sharp implements such as hair-grips, in an attempt to clean the ear; syringing or unskilled attempts to remove wax or foreign bodies may also be to blame.

Indirect trauma is usually caused by pressure from a slap with an open hand or from blast injury; it may occur from temporal bone fracture in a severe head injury. Welding sparks may cause burns to the tympanic membrane.

Symptoms

1 Pain, acute at time of rupture, usually transient.
2 Deafness, not usually severe, conductive in type. The cochlea may be injured if the stapes is driven into the inner ear in which case there is sensorineural deafness. Check the hearing and do the tuning forks tests.
3 Tinnitus may be persistent — this is cochlear damage.
4 Vertigo (rare).

Signs

1 Bleeding from the ear.
2 Blood clot in the ear canal.
3 A tear in the tympanic membrane (Fig. 7.1).

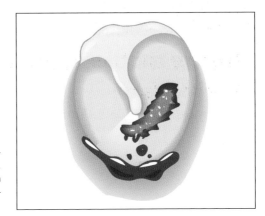

Figure 7.1 Traumatic perforation of the tympanic membrane, showing a ragged perforation with blood in the external auditory canal.

Treatment: leave it alone

1 Do *not* clean out the ear.
2 Do *not* put in drops.
3 Do *not* syringe.
4 Give antibiotics if there is evidence of infection.
5 Arrange careful surveillance until the hearing has returned to normal.

Clinical practice point

- Most traumatic perforations of the eardrum heal with no long-term adverse effects.

Chapter 8

Otitis media

Otitis media is inflammation of the middle ear. The term includes several different disease entities. A good understanding of terms is essential.

Acute otitis media

Acute otitis media (AOM) is a short-lived (usually 1–5 days) infection of the middle ear. If it is viral it may last as little as a day or so but it can persist causing pus to accumulate under pressure behind the eardrum, which may perforate. Before the eardrum perforates, AOM is intensely painful. It mainly occurs in children (Fig. 8.1).

Recurrent otitis media (ROM) refers to repeated such episodes, typically more than three in a 6-month period.

Otitis media with effusion

Otitis media with effusion (OME) is also common in children. Fluid – often thick sticky 'glue' – accumulates in the middle ear behind an intact drum. Because some fluid in the middle ear is normal for up to several weeks after an episode of AOM, the term OME requires that the fluid be persistent for at least 3 months.

Chronic otitis media

This implies that the eardrum has perforated, the perforation has failed to heal and there is ongoing infection. The term chronic suppurative otitis media

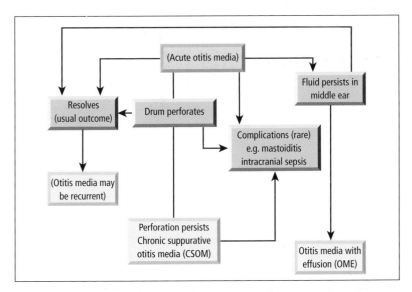

Figure 8.1 Algorithm to show outcomes of AOM.

(CSOM) is often used to emphasize the tendency for ears with longstanding perforations to become infected and discharge.

Cholesteatoma

Cholesteatoma is the accumulation of squamous epithelium in the middle ear, usually in an ear with a longstanding perforation. This is the most serious form of CSOM.

Clinical practice point

• 'Chronic otitis media' implies that the eardrum has perforated.

Chapter 9

Acute otitis media

Acute otitis media is common and frequently bilateral. Most children will develop one or more episodes typically before they are 2 years old.

It can follow an acute upper respiratory tract infection and may be viral or bacterial. A viral infection is short-lived (1 or 2 days) and often accompanied by some general features of an upper respiratory infection, e.g. pharyngitis and a runny nose.

Symptoms

Earache

Earache (otalgia) may be slight in a mild case, but more usually it is throbbing and severe. The child may cry and scream inconsolably until the ear perforates, the pain is relieved and peace is restored.

Deafness

Deafness is always present in acute otitis media. It is conductive in nature and may be accompanied by tinnitus. In an adult deafness or tinnitus may be the first complaint.

Signs

Pyrexia

The child is flushed and ill. The temperature may be as high as 40°C.

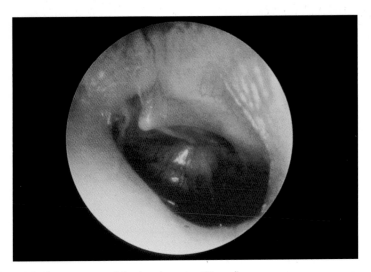

Figure 9.1 The appearance of the drum in acute otitis media.

Tenderness

There is usually some tenderness to pressure on the mastoid bone.

The tympanic membrane

The tympanic membrane varies in appearance according to the stage of the infection (Fig. 9.1). In early infection the drum is red, it becomes tense and bulging and may perforate with discharge of pus. Mucoid (sticky) discharge from an ear must mean that there is a perforation of the tympanic membrane. There are no mucous glands in the external canal. Otoscopy and interpreting the findings can be difficult in a fractious child.

Pathology

Acute otitis media is an infection of the mucous membrane of the whole of the middle-ear cleft – Eustachian tube, tympanic cavity, mastoid air cells.

The bacteria responsible for acute otitis media are: *Streptococcus pneumoniae* 35%, *Haemophilus influenzae* 25%, *Moraxella catarrhalis* 15%. Group A streptococci and *Staphylococcus aureus* may also be responsible.

The sequence of events in acute otitis media is as follows:

1 Organisms invade the mucous membrane causing inflammation, oedema, exudate, and later pus.

2 Oedema closes the Eustachian tube, preventing aeration and drainage.

3 Pressure from the pus rises, causing the drum to bulge and perforate.

4 Most cases resolve completely. A small number cause complications (see Chapter 11) or persistent perforation.

Treatment

Analgesics

Adequate analgesia is essential. Otitis media is painful and causes much misery. Simple analgesics, such as aspirin or paracetamol, should suffice but use adequate doses. Avoid the use of aspirin in children because of the risk of Reye's syndrome.

Antibiotics

Antibiotics are commonly prescribed but critics point out that they should be withheld at least in the early stages as the great majority of cases are self-limiting, and often viral. Widespread antibiotic use promotes the development of bacterial resistance. Some GPs give a prescription which the parents only need to get if the child doesn't improve in a day or so (Safety Net Antibiotic Prescription or 'SNAP'). A mild viral infection can be managed in this way but remember that otitis media is still a serious disease with potentially devastating complications. Make sure you are able to see the child for review and if in any doubt don't hesitate to use antibiotics. Penicillin or cephalosporins such as cefaclor remain the drugs of choice in most cases. There is no need for expensive third and fourth generation cephalosporins in the treatment of uncomplicated otits media.

Myringotomy

This is the creation of a small perforation in the eardrum – very rarely necessary – when bulging of the tympanic membrane persists, despite *adequate* antibiotic therapy or if there are complications. It should be carried out under general anaesthesia in theatre by an ENT surgeon. The ear may already be discharging when the patient is first seen – *nature's myringotomy*.

Further management

Acute otitis media is not cured until the hearing and the appearance of the membrane have returned to normal.

If there is no resolution suspect:

1 The nose, sinuses or nasopharynx. Infection may be present.
2 Low-grade infection in the mastoid cells.

Recurrent acute otitis media

Some children are susceptible to repeated attacks of acute otitis media. This causes a lot of distress to parents and children but usually resolves as the child gets older. Breast-feeding and avoidance of passive smoking help protect children. Very rarely there may be an underlying immunological deficit that will need to be investigated. If the attacks persist, grommet insertion or long-term treatment with low-dose antibiotics may prevent further attacks.

Clinical practice points

- Eardrops are of no value in acute otitis media with an intact drum.
- Adequate analgesia is essential.
- If antibiotics are withheld, make sure you can review the child after 24 h.
- Passive smoking predisposes children to otitis media.

Chapter 10

Chronic otitis media

Following an attack of acute otitis the perforation and discharge may persist – chronic otitis media. This leads to mixed infection and further damage to the middle-ear structures, with worsening conductive deafness. The predisposing factors in the development of chronic otitis media are listed in Box 10.1. Suppuration with discharge – chronic suppurative otitis media (CSOM) – can be further classified as in Box 10.2.

Box 10.1   Causes of chronic otitis media

1 Late or inadequate treatment of acute otitis media.
2 Upper airway sepsis.
3 Lowered resistance, e.g. malnutrition, anaemia, immunological impairment.
4 Particularly virulent infection, e.g. measles.

Box 10.2   Types of CSOM

1 *Mucosal disease* with tympanic membrane perforation (relatively safe).
2 *Bony:*
   (a) Osteitis.
   (b) Cholesteatoma – an epithelial sac which erodes the middle ear and adjacent structures including the meninges.

The perforated ear

A perforated eardrum may be asymptomatic. If unilateral, the relatively minor conductive hearing loss causes little or no trouble. The ear may discharge during an upper respiratory infection or if it becomes contaminated by water, e.g. after swimming. Some patients have persistent **mucosal infection (active CSOM)**. In

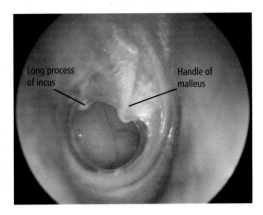

Figure 10.1 A large central perforation of the tympanic membrane. The handle of the malleus and the long process of the incus are visible (courtesy of MPJ Yardley).

these cases there may be underlying nasal or pharyngeal sepsis that will require attention if the ear is to heal. The ear will discharge, usually copiously, and the discharge is mucoid. The perforation may be large (Fig. 10.1) or very small and difficult to see. A short course of antibiotic eardrops can help dry up a discharging ear but many proprietary preparations contain aminoglycosides which can cause deafness. Ciprofloxacin is better. Systemic antibiotics are of little use. There is no point in persisting with prolonged courses of topical antibiotics. The mainstay of treatment is thorough and regular aural toilet. A small perforation may heal. Persistent infection can cause erosion of bone (**bony CSOM**) and eventually infection can spread beyond the ear, e.g. intracranial. Serious complications are very rare but if left untreated the condition may result in permanent deafness or intracranial sepsis. If squamous epithelium collects in the middle ear (**cholesteatoma**) it can erode adjacent structures and cause serious complications. Surgical repair may be necessary, especially if there is bony disease or cholesteatoma.

Myringoplasty

When there is a dry perforation, surgery may be considered but is *not mandatory*. *Myringoplasty* is the repair of a tympanic membrane perforation; various tissues have been used for graft material but that in most common use is autologous temporalis fascia, which is taken from just above the patient's ear. Success rates for this procedure are very high.

'Bony' CSOM or cholesteatoma

The bone affected by this type of CSOM comprises the tympanic ring, the ossicles, the mastoid air cells and the bony walls of the attic, aditus and antrum.

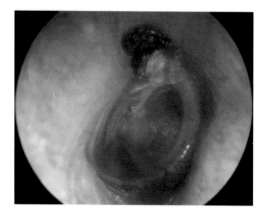

Figure 10.2 Crusting of the pars flaccida suggestive of underlying cholesteatoma (courtesy of MPJ Yardley).

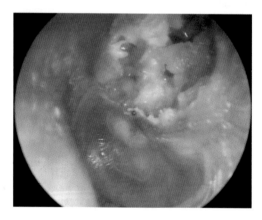

Figure 10.3 Erosion of the attic bone to reveal cholesteatoma (courtesy of MPJ Yardley).

The perforation is postero-superior (Fig. 10.2) or in the pars flaccida (Schrapnell's membrane) (Fig. 10.3). The discharge is often scanty but usually persistent, and may be foul smelling.

There are other features of this type of CSOM:

1 Granulations as a result of osteitis – bright red and bleed on touch.

2 Aural polyps formed of granulation tissue, which may fill the meatus and present at its outer end.

3 Cholesteatoma. This is formed by squamous epithelium within the middle ear. It results in accumulation of keratotic debris. This will be visible through the perforation as keratin flakes, which are white and smelly. The cholesteatoma expands and damages vital structures, such as dura, the facial nerve and the semicircular canals. *Cholesteatoma is potentially lethal if untreated.*

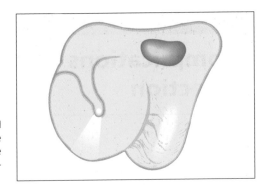

Figure 10.4 Modified radical mastoidectomy; note the shape of the cavity and the bulge caused by the lateral semicircular canal (blue).

Treatment of bony-type CSOM

1 **Regular aural toilet** in early cases of annular osteitis may be adequate to prevent progression, but such a case should be watched closely.

2 **Suction toilet** under the microscope may evacuate a small pocket of cholesteatoma, and a dry ear may result.

3 **Mastoidectomy** is nearly always necessary in established cholesteatoma. This is a major operation to open the mastoid cells, removing cholesteatoma and diseased tissue in the middle ear and mastoid (Fig. 10.4)

Clinical practice points

- An uncomplicated perforation may need no treatment.
- The mainstay of treatment is for a discharging ear is thorough and regular aural toilet.
- Cholesteatoma is potentially lethal if untreated.

Treatment

When the diagnosis of acute mastoiditis has been made, do not delay. The patient should be admitted to hospital.

• **Intravenous** antibiotics. If the organism is not known start amoxycillin and metronidazole immediately.

• **Surgery.** If there is a subperiosteal abscess or if the response to antibiotics is not rapid and complete, the pus needs to be drained under anaesthesia.

Facial paralysis

Facial paralysis can result from both acute and chronic otitis media.

1 Acute otitis media – especially in children and especially if the facial nerve canal in the middle ear is dehiscent. It is, however, uncommon. The prognosis for complete recovery is excellent.

2 Chronic otitis media – cholesteatoma may erode the bone around the facial nerve, and infection and granulations can cause facial paralysis.

Treatment

• If due to acute otitis media, a full recovery is to be expected with antibiotics.

• If due to chronic suppurative otitis media (CSOM), mastoidectomy is required with clearance of disease from around the facial nerve.

• Facial palsy in the presence of chronic ear disease is not Bell's palsy and active treatment is needed if the palsy is not to become permanent. *Do not give steroids.*

Labyrinthitis

Infection can spread from the middle ear to the cochlea but the inner ear is very well protected in its bony covering and this is a rare event. Infection may reach the labyrinth by erosion of a fistula by cholesteatoma. This can cause severe dizziness and sensorineural deafness.

Intracranial complications of otitis media

These arise when infection spreads from the ear into and beyond the meninges (Fig. 11.3). A number of clinical scenarios may ensue, i.e. meningitis, extradural abscess, brain abscess, subdural abscess, venous sinus thrombosis.

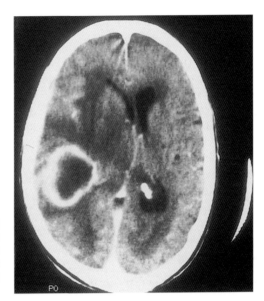

Figure 11.3 Computerized Tomography (CT) scan with contrast showing temporal lobe abscess resulting from chronic middle ear disease (courtesy of Dr T. Hodgson).

Meningitis

Clinical features

1 The patient is unwell.
2 Pyrexia – may only be slight.
3 Neck rigidity.
4 Positive Kernig's sign.
5 Photophobia.
Cerebrospinal fluid (CSF) – lumbar puncture essential unless there is raised intracranial pressure (q.v.).

Brain abscess

Otogenic brain abscess may occur in the cerebellum or in the temporal lobe of the cerebrum. The two routes by which infection reaches the brain are direct spread via bone and meninges or via blood vessels, i.e. thrombophlebitis.

A brain abscess may develop with great speed or more gradually over a period of months. The effects are produced by:

1 Systemic effects of infection, i.e. malaise, pyrexia – which may be absent;
2 Raised intracranial pressure, i.e. headache, drowsiness, confusion, impaired consciousness, papilloedema;
3 Focal signs, depending on where the abscess is, e.g. hemiparesis.

Diagnosis of intracranial sepsis

1 Any patient with chronic ear disease who develops headache, neurological signs or any of the features of meningitis – e.g. neck stiffness or photophobia – should be suspected of having intracranial extension.

2 Any patient who has otogenic meningitis, labyrinthitis or lateral sinus thrombosis may have a brain abscess as well.

3 Lumbar puncture may be dangerous owing to pressure coning but is the best way to confirm meningitis. Seek expert advice.

4 Seek neurosurgical advice early if you suspect intracranial suppuration.

5 Confirmation and localization of the abscess will require further investigation. Computerized tomography (CT) scanning will demonstrate intracranial abscesses reliably. Magnetic resonance (MR) imaging shows soft-tissue lesions with more detail than CT but gives no bone detail. If in doubt what to do, discuss the problem with a radiologist.

Treatment

It is the brain abscess that will kill the patient, and this must take surgical priority. The abscess should be drained through a burr hole, or excised via a craniotomy. Then, if the patient's condition permits, mastoidectomy should be performed under the same anaesthetic. After pus has been obtained for culture, aggressive therapy with antibiotics is essential, to be amended as necessary when the sensitivity is known.

Prognosis

The prognosis of brain abscess has improved with the use of antibiotics and modern diagnostic methods but still carries a high mortality; the outlook is better for cerebral abscesses than cerebellar, in which the mortality rate may be 70%. Left untreated, death from brain abscess occurs from pressure coning, rupture into a ventricle or spreading encephalitis. Patients who recover may be left with hemiparesis or epilepsy.

Clinical practice point

- Otitis media is still a potentially lethal disease. Intracranial complications can be fatal.

Chapter 12

Otitis media with effusion

Childhood otitis media with effusion

Following an episode of otitis media many children will be slightly deaf for several weeks. This is due to an accumulation of fluid in the middle ear. Sometimes fluid accumulates without a prior episode of acute otitis media – a middle ear effusion. Provided this is short-lived and resolves completely it is a normal part of childhood and needs no treatment. If fluid persists in the middle ear with an intact drum, i.e. no perforation, for a continuous period of 3 months or more this is pathological and is termed 'otitis media with effusion' (OME), or 'glue ear'. 'Serous otitis media' and 'secretory otitis media' are older descriptive terms still often used for this condition. Avoid calling this 'chronic' as the term 'chronic otitis media' is best reserved for conditions in which the eardrum has perforated.

Prevalence

Fluid in the middle ear affects most children at one time or another. In up to a third of children it is at some time in their childhood persistent for 3 months or more (OME). OME is commoner in the winter. It is commonest in small children and those of primary school age and may cause significant deafness. It may be responsible for developmental and educational impairment, and if untreated may result in permanent middle-ear changes.

Aetiology

Many cases of OME follow an acute otitis media and are due to persistence of fluid after the acute infection has subsided. In other cases the aetiology is

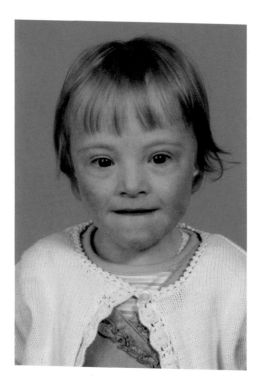

Figure 12.1 Child with Down Syndrome.

unknown. The **adenoids** have an important role. Adenoidectomy can be curative in some cases of OME. Large adenoids can obstruct the Eustachian tube so that the middle ear is poorly ventilated and fluid accumulates. The adenoids may also act as a reservoir for clumps of bacteria, which are encased in a polysaccharide matrix and resistant to treatment with antibiotics or to the normal physiological defence mechanisms (a '*Biofilm*').

Passive smoking, nasal allergy, and **early exposure to pathogens** such as occurs in crèches and day-care facilities for groups of young children have all been implicated in OME.

Cleft palate children are especially susceptible to OME. This is due to palatal muscle dysfunction, which affects the Eustachian tube. Children with **Down Syndrome** (Fig. 12.1) and with **mucociliary function disorders** are also at increased risk.

Presentation and effects

Fluid in the middle ear interferes with transmission of sound so a conductive deafness ensues. This is rarely severe – about 30 decibels is usual – and children

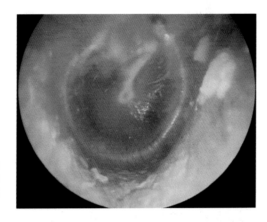

Figure 12.2 OME. Note the yellow discoloration of the tympanic membrane (courtesy of MPJ Yardley).

can often manage very well. If it is persistent and bilateral it will cause noticeable problems – often enough to affect adversely the child's school performance. Parents complain that the child won't come when called, turns the television up loud, shouts and becomes easily frustrated and bad-tempered. There is no pain, but some parents notice that the child is clumsy and unsteady. Otoscopy will often show the characteristic dull yellowish appearance of fluid behind the drum but findings can be difficult to interpret especially in young children (Fig. 12.2). An audiogram or hearing test confirms the conductive deafness. In children under four, pure tone audiometry is difficult and unreliable but an experienced and trained tester will usually be able to get a good estimate of the child's hearing thresholds by other methods, e.g. observing the child's behaviour in response to sound stimuli. Impedance audiometry (Chapter 2) is helpful to show the 'flat curve' typical of fluid in the middle ear.

Management of OME

Many children will **improve spontaneously**. GPs will often try a single course of antibiotics to help shift an established effusion but there is little point in persisting with repeated antibiotics. If there is a **predisposing condition**, e.g. allergic rhinitis, upper respiratory sepsis or cleft palate – this may need treatment on its own merits. Treatment of OME is mainly geared toward improving the hearing. The traditional approach has been the insertion of a small tube in the eardrum (**grommet**, Fig. 12.3). This is done under a general anaesthetic following puncture of the drum and aspiration of the fluid (myringotomy). The grommet now permits air entry into the middle ear, which stops re-accumulation of fluid. Hence grommets are sometimes referred to as ventilation tubes or 'vents'.

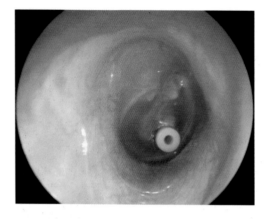

Figure 12.3 Right tympanic membrane with grommet in place (courtesy of MPJ Yardley).

Most 'vents' will extrude after a period of up to 1 year and the child needs no further treatment. Grommets or 'vents' are effective but associated with some morbidity, e.g. the risk of persistent perforation of the drum (about 5%) and of infection and discharge due to what amounts to a perforation of the drum while the grommets are in place.

Adenoidectomy is effective but can be complicated by bleeding. Some ENT surgeons combine grommets with adenoidectomy, especially in children with recurrent effusions or where there is evidence of adenoid hypertrophy, e.g. upper airway obstruction.

Many parents and doctors are concerned about the complications of grommets and prefer to encourage the child to use a **hearing aid** for a period of several months to a year or so while the middle ear effusions resolve spontaneously. In addition to conventional hearing aids a simple amplification device that the child can wear on a headband (e.g. 'Softband', Fig. 12.4) may suffice in cases where the hearing loss is mild.

Adult OME

OME in adults usually follows an upper respiratory infection. Improvement is gradual and spontaneous, but may take up to 6 weeks. A nasal decongestant – for a short period – may hasten resolution. An effusion can also follow sudden changes in ear pressure – e.g. deep sea diving or rapid descent in an aircraft (barotrauma), can persist after an episode of acute otitis media as in children or may be a sign of Eustachian tube obstruction. Rarely it can be a presentation of

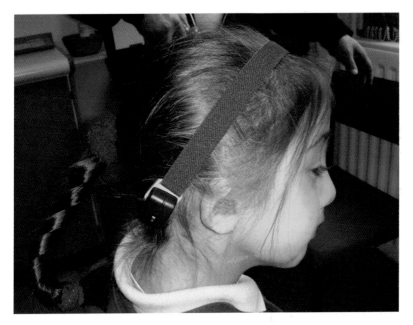

Figure 12.4 Child using 'Softband' amplifier.

nasopharyngeal malignancy. If there is no obvious explanation such as barotrauma or a recent ear infection examination of the nasopharynx to exclude tumour is essential.

Clinical practice points

• Fluid in the middle ear is a normal event in childhood. It only needs treatment if it is persistent and causes deafness.

• Think of a nasopharyngeal tumour in an adult with an unexplained middle ear effusion.

Chapter 13

Otosclerosis

Otosclerosis causes abnormal bone to be formed around the stapes footplate, preventing its normal movement. Conductive deafness results. It is commoner in women, typically presents in early adult life and often progresses during pregnancy. There may be a family history. Apart from conductive deafness, evident on tuning fork tests (Chapter 3), examination is typically normal. More rarely, the bone of the cochlea is affected and results in sensorineural deafness.

Treatment

Hearing aids

Modern hearing aids are of great benefit to patients with conductive deafness. They have the advantage of causing no risk to the patient's hearing. A hearing aid should always be offered to a patient as an alternative to surgery.

Stapedectomy

First performed in 1956, stapedectomy is an elegant solution to the problem. The middle ear is exposed (Fig. 13.1), the upper part of the stapes (stapes 'superstructure') is removed and the footplate perforated. A prosthesis of stainless steel or Teflon in place of the stapes is attached to the incus with its distal end in the 'oval window', a thin membrane which separates the middle and the inner ear (Fig. 13.2). Stapedectomy is a highly specialized procedure. There is a risk of total loss of hearing in the operated ear.

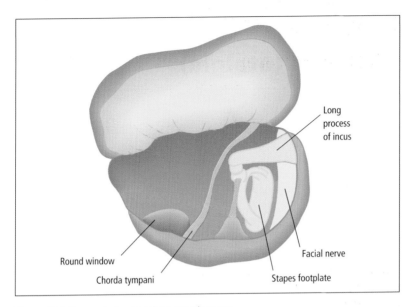

Figure 13.1 The surgical approach to stapedectomy.

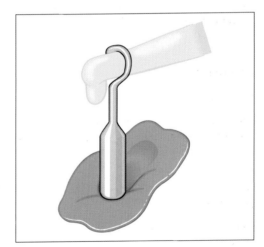

Figure 13.2 Stapedectomy. The superstructure of the stapes has been removed, the footplate opened and covered with a vein graft before inserting a prosthetic piston.

Clinical practice point

- In an adult with conductive deafness and a normal eardrum, think of otosclerosis.

Chapter 14

Earache (otalgia)

Earache may be due to ear disease (aural causes), or to disease elsewhere (referred earache).

Aural causes

The most common causes are *acute otitis media, acute otitis externa, furunculosis* and, very rarely, *acute mastoiditis*. Malignant disease of the ear may cause intractable earache.

Referred earache

In referred pain pathology in a structure supplied by a sensory nerve can cause pain to be felt in another structure supplied by that same nerve. The ear has a rich nerve supply and is especially susceptible. Figure 14.1 shows the sensory nerve supply of some of the structures of the head and neck and helps to explain why referred earache is so common. Examples of structures that cause earache due to referred pain are:

- Carious teeth, impacted molar teeth, the temporomandibular joint or the tongue (trigeminal nerve, auriculo-temporal branch).
- The tonsil and the tongue base (glossopharyngeal nerve). Earache can be very severe after tonsillectomy.
- The larynx or pharynx.
- The neck (great auricular and lesser occipital nerves).

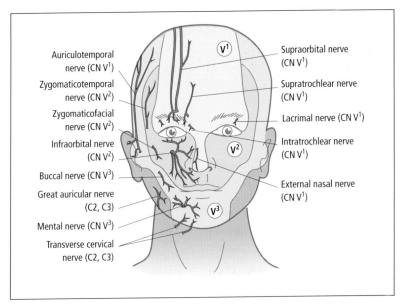

Figure 14.1 Sensory nerve supply of the head and neck. V1, V2 and V3: first, second and third divisions of the trigeminal nerve; CN: cranial nerve; C: cervical nerve.

Clinical practice point

- If the ear is normal on examination, look for a source of referred pain.

Chapter 15

Tinnitus

Box 15.1   Local and general causes of tinnitus

Local causes

Tinnitus may be a symptom of any abnormal condition of the ear and may be associated with any form of deafness.
- Presbycusis – often causes tinnitus.
- Menière's disease – tinnitus is usually worse with the acute attacks.
- Noise-induced deafness – tinnitus may be worse immediately after exposure to noise.
- Aneurysm, vascular malformation and some vascular intracranial tumours, e.g. glomus jugulare tumour can cause 'pulsatile' tinnitus, which may even be heard by an examiner. Listen to the side of the head with a stethoscope.

General causes

Tinnitus is often a feature of general ill-health as in:
- Fever.
- Cardiovascular disease – hypertension, atheroma, cardiac failure.
- Blood disease – anaemia, raised viscosity.
- Neurological disease – multiple sclerosis, neuropathy.
- Drug treatment – aspirin, quinine, ototoxic drugs.
- Alcohol abuse.

Tinnitus is the complaint of noises in the ears in the absence of a sound stimulus. It is not a disease but a symptom. Most people experience transient tinnitus at some time, particularly after exposure to loud noise. The exact cause is unknown but it is thought to be due to inappropriate activity in the hair cells of the cochlea. There are multiple possible causes but most cases are idiopathic (see Box 15.1). It is especially common in diseases such as presbycusis which affect hair cell function. It can be a very unwelcome feature of advancing age. Most tinnitus patients notice that the noises are worse in quiet surroundings. Tinnitus is aggravated by fatigue, anxiety and depression.

Management

The management of a patient with tinnitus is a severe test of a doctor's art. Management focuses on excluding treatable causes and helping patients cope.

Tinnitus due to chronic degeneration, such as presbycusis, ototoxicity or noise-induced deafness, is usually permanent. With time, the tinnitus will obtrude less as the patient adjusts to it and avoids circumstances that aggravate it. It very rarely goes away completely.

Take the patient's fears and complaints seriously. Take a thorough history and examine the patient properly. Many patients fear that tinnitus indicates serious disease of the ear or a brain tumour. A quick look at the tympanic membranes is only a gesture. Reassurance will be more credible if examination has been adequate. Always test the hearing. If you find an abnormality of the ear such as impacted wax or otitis media, treatment will often cure the tinnitus.

Patients with depression are particularly susceptible to the effects of tinnitus. Severe tinnitus may precipitate depression – treat it expertly, thoroughly and sympathetically.

Drug treatment, such as sedatives and antidepressants, may help the patient but will not eliminate tinnitus. Anticonvulsant drugs and vasodilators may be of benefit but their effectiveness cannot be predicted.

If the patient with tinnitus is also deaf, a hearing aid is very helpful not only to rehabilitate the hearing loss but in 'masking' the tinnitus.

'Tinnitus maskers' or 'white noise generators' will also make tinnitus less obtrusive. A typical device looks like a postural hearing aid and its output characteristics can be adjusted to obtain the most effective frequency and intensity.

If the patient is kept awake by tinnitus, a radio with a time switch may help. Many patients use a 'pillow masker' obtainable in most electrical stores, which emits a constant low intensity sound that helps patients to focus on a sound other than the tinnitus that is often easier to tolerate.

Many patients use relaxation techniques, acupuncture and herbal remedies.

Patients will often read of new 'cures' for tinnitus in the popular press. Sadly these will almost always prove useless and cause more distress and disappointment when it transpires they don't work.

Patients who are very distressed may find counselling by a skilled hearing therapist helpful.

It is helpful for patients to understand that this is an extremely common problem and the British Tinnitus Association website (www.tinnitus.org.uk) can be a useful resource.

Clinical practice points

- Tinnitus can be an extremely distressing complaint. Treat it and the patient seriously.
- Most cases are idiopathic.
- Beware supposed new 'cures' for tinnitus.

Chapter 16

Balance disorders

Applied physiology

The physiology of balance is complex. The body's sense of equilibrium is maintained by input from a number of sources. These include the eyes, proprioceptive organs especially in the muscles and joints of the neck, peripheral nerves, the labyrinth or 'balance organ' in the inner ear which includes the *vestibule* and *semicircular canals* and the cerebral cortex and cerebellum. Input from all these sources converges in the brain stem; dysfunction of any of these systems may lead to imbalance, a feeling of unsteadiness, 'vertigo' – a sensation of movement – and a tendency to fall. Vertigo may be accompanied by 'nystagmus' – a rapid beating of the eyes to one side as impulses from the brain stem to the ocular muscles attempt to correct the patient's balance. Balance disorders are common, particularly in the elderly. They can be extremely disabling, restricting patients' ability to look after themselves and causing great distress. Patients often believe they have developed a serious and incurable disease. Happily most cases are due to benign and often self-limiting pathology.

Diagnosis

Some of the main causes are listed in Table 16.1. The diagnosis of the cause of vertigo or imbalance depends mostly on history, much on examination and little on investigation. Patients can mean very different things by terms such as 'dizziness', 'funny turns', 'vertigo' and 'loss of balance'. Take a careful and meticulous history. Pay particular attention to *timing*, i.e. are the symptoms constant or episodic; are they short-lived as in the few minutes of dizziness associated with benign positional vertigo, or do they last for a few hours as in Menière's disease;

Table 16.1 Guide to causes of vertigo

Episodic with ear symptoms
- Migraine
- Menière's disease

Episodic without ear symptoms
- Migraine
- Benign paroxysmal positional vertigo
- Transient ischaemic attacks
- Epilepsy
- Cardiac dysrhythmia
- Postural hypotension
- Cervical spondylosis

Constant with ear symptoms
- Chronic otitis media with labyrinthine fistula
- Ototoxicity
- Acoustic neuroma

Constant without aural symptoms
- Multiple sclerosis
- Intracranial tumour
- Cardiovascular disease
- Degenerative disorder of the vestibular labyrinth
- Hyperventilation
- Alcoholism

Solitary acute attack with ear symptoms
- Viral infection, e.g. mumps, herpes zoster
- Vascular occlusion
- Labyrinthine fistula
- Round-window membrane rupture/head injury

Solitary acute attack without aural symptoms
- Acute labyrinthitis
- Vasovagal faint
- Vestibular neuronitis
- Trauma

are there associated *ear symptoms*, e.g. deafness, tinnitus, earache or discharge; and are there *neurological* features, i.e. loss of consciousness, weakness, numbness, dysarthria and diplopia, or seizures. Note the *past medical history* and make a record of the patient's *medications*. The cause of balance disorders can be multi-factorial, especially in the elderly.

Common specific disorders

Benign paroxysmal positional vertigo

In benign paroxysmal positional vertigo (BPPV) short-lived (often a few seconds) attacks of vertigo are precipitated by turning the head, especially when the patient is in bed. A sensation that the head is 'spinning' occurs following a latent period of several seconds. This is thought to be due to a degenerative condition of the utricle of the inner ear which causes calcified particles to shear off the highly specialized neuro-epithelium. BPPV may occur spontaneously or following head injury. It is also seen in chronic otitis media. The symptoms can be reproduced by rapidly turning the patient's head while she is lying on an examination couch with her head gently lowered below the head of the couch and supported firmly by the examiner, (Hallpike Positional Manoeuvre). Nystagmus will be seen but repeated testing results in abolition of the vertigo. Steady resolution of BPPV is to be expected over a period of weeks or months. It may be recurrent.

Treatment

BPPV can often be relieved completely by the Epley or 'particle repositioning' manoeuvre. This is a series of sequential controlled movements of the head usually carried out by a skilled audiologist which is said to work by dislodging calcified particles ('otoliths') within the inner ear fluids.

Menière's disease

Menière's disease is fortunately uncommon, but may be incapacitating. This is a condition of unknown aetiology but interest has focused on distension of the structures in the inner ear by retained fluid. There is a typical triad of symptoms, of vertigo, deafness and tinnitus. The attacks can last from a few hours to several days. Vomiting is common during attacks. It can occur at any age, but its onset is most common between 40 and 60 years. It usually starts in one ear, but the second becomes affected in 25% of cases. Although deafness is fluctuant repeated attacks can cause significant sensorineural hearing loss. Tinnitus may be constant but is more severe before an attack.

Treatment

Medical

Anti-emetics and labyrinthine sedatives are helpful in an acute attack, but when vomiting is likely to occur oral medication is of limited value. Cinnarizine and prochlorperazine are useful. Prochlorperazine can be given as a suppository or sublabially, or chlorpromazine may be given as an intramuscular injection. Between attacks, various methods of treatment are used but the evidence for their efficacy is weak. They include:

- Fluid and salt restriction.
- Avoidance of smoking and excessive alcohol or coffee.
- Regular therapy with betahistine hydrochloride.
- Labyrinthine sedatives, e.g. cinnarizine or prochlorperazine.
- Low-dose diuretic therapy.

Surgical

Some ENT surgeons will offer surgery for patients with severe disabling Menière's disease which cannot be controlled by the above measures. Techniques include labyrinthectomy but as this destroys the hearing it is only considered in unilateral cases and when the hearing is already severely impaired. An alternative is the instillation of an ototoxic drug such as gentamycin into the inner ear. There is a significant risk to hearing with this technique. Surgical division of the vestibular nerve preserves the hearing but is a hazardous procedure.

Vertebrobasilar insufficiency

Ischaemia in the part of the brain supplied by the vertebrobasilar artery can cause momentary attacks of vertigo. These are typically precipitated by neck extension, e.g. hanging washing on a line. The diagnosis is more certain if other features of brain stem ischaemia such as dysarthria or diplopia, are present. Severe ischaemia may cause 'drop attacks' without loss of consciousness.

Ototoxic drugs

Ototoxic drugs, such as gentamycin and other aminoglycoside antibiotics, can cause disabling and permanent loss of balance by destruction of labyrinthine function. The risk is reduced by careful monitoring of serum levels of the drug, especially in patients with renal impairment. There is not usually any rotational vertigo, just a sensation of poor balance control (ataxia).

Acute labyrinthitis

Acute suppurative or pyogenic labyrinthitis causes severe vertigo and total loss of hearing. This can complicate otitis media. The term 'acute labyrinthitis' is also used to describe a sudden onset of vertigo of unknown aetiology associated with vomiting and in severe cases collapse. Nystagmus is a prominent feature. The structures in the labyrinth include both the vestibule, which is concerned with balance and the cochlea. If the hearing is unaffected it is assumed that rather than affecting the entire labyrinth the cochlea is spared and the term vestibular neuronitis is used. A viral cause is often assumed. Some cases may be due to a vascular event. To emphasize the uncertainty over aetiology many authors prefer the term 'acute vestibular failure' or 'recurrent vestibulopathy'. Management is similar to that of Meniere's disease in the acute phase. Improvement takes place over a period of weeks and is quicker in younger patients. There may be residual imbalance which can take months or years to resolve.

Trauma to the labyrinth

Trauma to the labyrinth causing vertigo may complicate head injury, with or without temporal bone fracture. Vertigo may occur after ear surgery and will usually settle in a few days.

Clinical practice point

• Acute loss of balance is extremely frightening. Many patients will suspect they have developed a brain tumour or some serious disease but most of the causes of balance disorders are benign.

Chapter 17

Facial nerve paralysis

Applied anatomy and physiology

The facial (**seventh cranial, VII**) nerve provides motor fibres to the muscles of facial expression. It originates in the seventh nerve nucleus in the brain stem (pons), enters the middle ear and mastoid and exits the skull at the stylomastoid foramen just in front of the mastoid process. From here it enters the parotid gland where it divides into its branches (Fig. 17.1). Paralysis can be caused by pathology anywhere along the nerve course or in the cortical nerves which

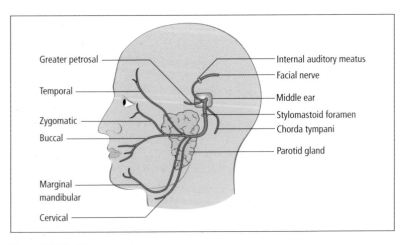

Greater petrosal

Temporal

Zygomatic

Buccal

Marginal mandibular

Cervical

Internal auditory meatus

Facial nerve

Middle ear

Stylomastoid foramen

Chorda tympani

Parotid gland

Figure 17.1 Facial nerve anatomy.

Table 17.1 Common causes of facial nerve paralysis

Supranuclear and nuclear (upper motor neurone)
- Vascular lesions, e.g. stroke
- Intracranial tumours
- Multiple sclerosis

Infranuclear (lower motor neurone)
- 'Bell's palsy'
- Trauma (birth injury, fractured temporal bone, surgical)
- Tumours (parotid tumours, acoustic neuroma, malignant disease of the middle ear)
- Middle ear suppuration (acute or chronic otitis media)
- 'Ramsay Hunt' syndrome
- Guillain–Barré syndrome
- Sarcoidosis

control the nucleus (supranuclear or upper motor neurone fibres) resulting in asymmetric movement of some or all of the muscles of facial expression. Facial nerve palsy causes difficulty with smiling, frowning and expressing emotions. It is a devastating condition for the patient. The causes are numerous and are considered in Table 17.1.

'Supranuclear' or upper motor neurone causes will often spare the forehead as these muscles receive fibres from both facial nerve nuclei.

Clinical diagnosis

The patient presents with weakness of the facial muscles, difficulty in clearing food from inside the cheek, or drooling from one side of the mouth. Facial asymmetry is accentuated by asking the patient to attempt to close the eyes tightly, show the teeth or whistle (Fig. 17.2).

Involuntary movements (e.g. smiling) may be retained even in the lower face. A careful history and aural and neurological examination are essential. Sparing of the forehead suggests a supranuclear pathology. Impaired taste implies the lesion is above the origin of the chorda tympani; reduction of tear production (lacrimation) suggests the lesion is above the geniculate ganglion where the superficial petrosal nerve arises (Fig. 17.1).

Bell's palsy (idiopathic facial paralysis)

Bell's palsy is a lower motor neurone facial palsy of unknown cause, but thought to be viral. Bell's palsy may be complete or incomplete; the more severe the

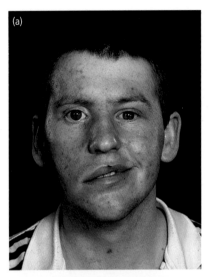

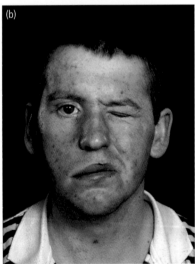

Figure 17.2 Post-traumatic right facial palsy. Shown at rest (a) and on attempted eye closure (b).

palsy, the worse the prognosis. In practice, full recovery may be expected in over 90% of cases. The remainder may develop persistent paraylsis and other complications including ectropion (weakness of the muscles of the lower eyelid causing persistent overflow of tears) or an aberrant sequence of movements of the face (synkinesis).

Management

Treatment of Bell's palsy should not be delayed. Prednisolone given orally is the treatment of choice, but it must commence in the first 24h. In an adult, start with 80mg daily and reduce the dose steadily to zero over 2 weeks. Be vigilant about eye care. The protective blink reflex may be lost and the cornea exposed, especially at night. An eye-pad, a tape over the eyelids at night or in persistent cases a 'tarsorrhaphy' (surgical approximation of the eyelids) may be needed. Persistent facial palsy warrants referral and thorough investigation, including CT or MRI scanning.

Electrodiagnosis is used in the assessment of the degree of involvement of the nerve and includes nerve conduction tests and electromyography. A detailed description of the various tests is beyond the scope of this book, but their application is of value as a guide to prognosis and management.

Ramsay Hunt syndrome

This is due to herpes zoster infection of the geniculate ganglion, affecting more rarely the glossopharyngeal (IX) and vagus (X) nerves and, very occasionally, the trigeminal (V), abducens (VI) or hypoglossal (XII) nerves. The patient is usually elderly, and severe pain precedes the facial palsy. The patient often has vertigo, and the hearing is impaired. The characteristic clinical feature is a vesicular eruption in the ear (sometimes on the tongue and palate). Recovery of facial nerve function is much less likely than in Bell's palsy.

Prompt treatment with acyclovir given orally may improve the prognosis and reduce post-herpetic neuralgia.

Clinical practice points

- Do not make a diagnosis of Bell's palsy until you have excluded other causes. If recovery does not commence in 6 weeks, reconsider the diagnosis.
- Facial palsy in acute or chronic otitis media requires immediate expert advice. Urgent surgical treatment may be needed.

Chapter 18

Clinical examination of the nose and nasopharynx

Illumination and inspection

The first requirement is adequate lighting. Ideally this is obtained with a head-light, an endoscope or a head-mirror to reflect light from an adjustable strong light source. All of these take some training and experience to use well. A bright torch or better still an auriscope with the largest speculum that will fit into the nasal cavity provides a good alternative (Fig. 18.1).

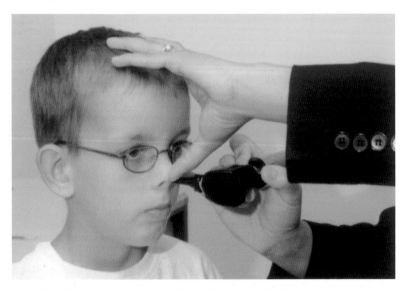

Figure 18.1 Using an aural speculum to inspect the nasal cavity. Note the direction of view.

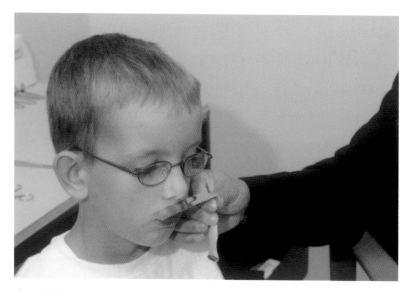

Figure 18.2 Assessing the nasal airway using a metal tongue depressor.

First inspect the exterior of the nose. Look for asymmetry of the nasal bones and gently lift the nasal tip to look for any deviation of the septum and any evidence of inflammation of the skin around the entrance to the nasal cavity (vestibule).

The nasal airway

Now assess the nasal airway. You can do this by gently occluding one nostril at a time and asking the patient to breathe in through the other side, or by holding a cool polished surface, such as a metal tongue depressor, below the nostrils. The area of condensation from each side of the nose can be compared.

Anterior rhinoscopy

Most students are unaware of the interior dimensions and relations of the nose, which extends horizontally backwards for 65–76mm to the posterior nasal apertures or 'choanae'. Remember that the interior of the nose is much more horizontal than most students think and that the nasal mucosa is very sensitive! When you look in remember to look 'back' rather than 'up' (Fig. 18.2). The inside of the nose may be obscured by mucosal oedema or septal deviations.

ENT surgeons will sometimes use a Thudicum's speculum (Fig. 18.3), which is introduced gently into the nose. In children, a speculum is often not necessary as an adequate view can be obtained by lifting the nasal tip with the thumb.

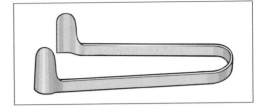

Figure 18.3 Thudicum's speculum.

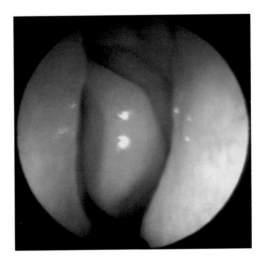

Figure 18.4 The appearance of the normal nose showing the inferior turbinate attached to the lateral nasal wall (courtesy of TJ Woolford).

On looking into the nose the anterior septum and inferior turbinates are easily seen (Fig. 18.4). It is a common error to mistake the turbinates for a nasal polyp. Turbinates are sensitive, and are attached to the lateral nasal wall. A polyp is often greyish, translucent and insensitive to touch.

Nasal endoscope

Rigid or fibre-optic endoscopes have made examination of the nose and nasopharynx much easier. The instrument is introduced through the nose and the post-nasal space can be inspected at leisure. It has the advantage of allowing photography and simultaneous viewing by an observer. It also allows minute inspection of the nasal cavity.

Clinical practice point

- An auriscope with a large speculum provides a good view of the inside of the nose. Practice makes perfect.

Chapter 19

Foreign body in the nose

Children sometimes insert foreign bodies into one or both nostrils (Fig. 19.1). The culprit may be the child or a schoolyard or nursery chum! The objects of their choice may be hard, such as buttons, beads or ball bearings, or soft, such as paper, cotton wool, rubber or other vegetable materials; the latter, being as a rule more irritating, tend to give rise to symptoms more quickly.

The child, however intelligent, is unlikely to indicate that a foreign body is present in his nose; he may, in fact, deny the possibility in order to avoid rebuke. A sibling may give the game away.

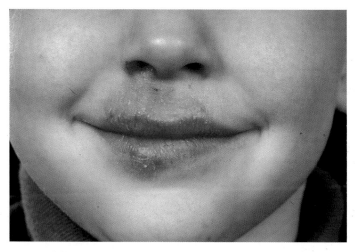

Figure 19.1 A child with a foreign body in the right nostril.

Clinical features

- A fretful child.
- Unilateral evil-smelling nasal discharge, sometimes blood-stained.
- Excoriation around the nostril (vestibulitis).
- Occasionally, X-ray evidence.

Dangers

- Injury from clumsy attempts at removal by unskilled persons.
- Local spread of infection – sinusitis or meningitis.
- Inhalation of foreign body – leading to lung collapse and infection. This is very rare.
- Nasal septal perforation – especially with 'button batteries'.

Management

Be alive to the possibility of nasal foreign bodies in small children. The child's mother may say that she suspects a foreign body, or the presence of a foreign body may be obvious. On the other hand, there is often an element of uncertainty, and full reassurance cannot be given until every step has been taken to reveal the true state of affairs. *When in doubt, call in expert advice.* In the case of a cooperative child it may be possible, with a head-mirror (or lamp) and Thudicum's speculum to see and, with small nasal forceps or blunt hooks, to remove the foreign body without general anaesthetic. Local analgesia and decongestion are helpful and may be applied in the form of a small cotton-wool swab wrung out in lidocaine/phenylephrine solution. Extreme care is necessary. A fractious child will need a general anaesthetic. This must be administered by an experienced anaesthetist, and it is usual to employ an endotracheal tube. The surgeon may then remove the foreign body and need to have no fear that it will enter the trachea. Rarely, an adult complaining of nasal obstruction is found to have a large concretion blocking one side of the nose. This is a rhinolith, and consists of many layers of calcium and magnesium salts that have formed around a small central nucleus. The latter often contains a foreign body.

Clinical practice points

- If a mother or carer suspects a nasal foreign body, do not reassure her until you have fully inspected both nasal cavities with a good light. This may need a general anaesthetic. If in doubt, seek help.
- A button battery is potentially dangerous as corrosive fluid may leak from it. It must be removed especially quickly.

Chapter 20

Injuries of the nose

Injury may cause:
- Bleeding.
- Injury to the nasal septum.
- Fractures of the nasal bones.

Fracture of the nasal bones (Fig. 20.1)

The fracture is often simple but can be comminuted with multiple fragments. There may be an open wound in the skin over the nasal bones – compound fracture.

Clinical features

- Bruising of the skin and subcutaneous tissues over the nasal bones.
- Tenderness over the fracture site.
- Mobility of the nose.
- Deformity, i.e. the shape of the nose has altered (not always present).

Treatment

The patient may have had multiple injuries and need resuscitation. Fractured noses usually bleed. Control this first. Examine carefully to make sure there are no other facial fractures, e.g. orbital rim, mandible. Lacerations should be cleaned meticulously to avoid tattooing with dirt and carefully repaired.

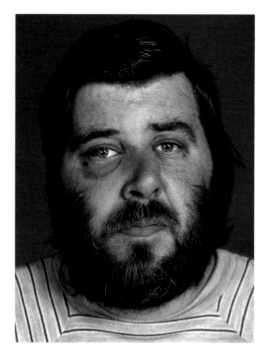

Figure 20.1 Patient with nasal fracture showing gross displacement of the nasal bones to the left and bruising below the right eye.

Septal haematoma

Sometimes, soon after a punch on the nose, the victim complains of very severe nasal obstruction. This may be caused by a septal haematoma – the result of bleeding between the two layers of muco-perichondrium covering the septum. It is often (but not always) associated with a fracture of the septum. The appearance is quite distinctive. Both nasal passages are obliterated by a boggy, pink or dull red swelling replacing the septum. Treatment may not be needed for a very small haematoma, but a large one requires incision along the base of the septum, evacuation of the clot, insertion of a drain and nasal packing to approximate the septal coverings of muco-perichondrium. Antibiotic cover should be considered to avert the development of a septal abscess. At worst this will cause 'saddling' of the nose as the cartilage necroses. The patient should be warned that there may be permanent deformity of the nose.

Dislocation of the nasal bones

This is far more common than a septal haematoma. If a previously straight nose is bent following an injury, it must be broken. If it is not bent after an injury, the bones will heal and there will be no external deformity. Stand behind and above the patient's head and look down on the nose. If there is no deformity, no manipulation or splinting is needed. If the nasal bones are displaced, plan a reduction of the fracture.

Septal dislocation

Nasal injury often results in deviation of the nasal septum, causing airway obstruction. This rarely needs immediate treatment. If there is no external deformity an ENT surgeon will arrange septal surgery – 'septoplasty' – after a period of weeks or months. If there is a complex injury to both the bones and the cartilage a good result may only be obtained by simultaneous correction of both – before the bones have set.

When to reduce the fracture

Nasal fractures can be reduced immediately after the injury by simple manipulation, but the appropriate medical attendant is rarely present. More often, the patient presents himself to the casualty officer some time later, by which time oedema may obscure the extent of any deformity and pain precludes manipulation. Oedema will settle over 5–7 days. Make sure the patient sees an ENT surgeon within a week of injury. After 2 weeks, the bone may be fixed and deformity may be permanent. The optimum timing for straightening the nose is usually 7–10 days after the injury.

Reduction of fractured nasal bones

Some units prefer general anaesthesia with endotracheal intubation. Nasal fractures are now increasingly dealt with in outpatients under local anaesthetic. The nasal mucosa is painted with local anaesthetic and a vasoconstrictor and the external nasal nerve at its exit below the nasal bone is blocked with lidocaine (lignocaine). Nasal bone manipulation can then be carried out with minimal discomfort. Depressed nasal fractures will require elevation with forceps. External splinting is rarely needed.

Late treatment of nasal fractures

If a patient with a fractured nose presents months or years after injury, manipulation is clearly not possible, and formal corrective surgery to both the bones and the cartilage – septorhinoplasty – is the only way to correct the deformity.

It is a difficult procedure and it is far better to treat a nasal fracture well at the time of injury.

Clinical practice points

- Check a patient with a nasal injury for other facial fractures.
- Look for a septal haematoma and if you suspect one refer immediately to ENT.
- Make sure nasal fractures are seen by an ENT surgeon within 7 days of the injury.
- X-rays are of doubtful value in nasal fractures. Decide whether the patient needs a reduction based on whether or not there is a visible external deformity.

Chapter 21

Epistaxis

Epistaxis (nasal bleeding) is common.

Applied basic science

The nose has a very rich blood supply. One of the functions of the nose is to warm and humidify inspired air. The nasal epithelium undergoes constant variation in the state of engorgement of its blood vessels. Vessels from both the internal and external carotid artery contribute to the nose, i.e. the ethmoidal arteries from the internal carotid and the greater palatine superior labial and sphenopalatine arteries from the external carotid. These vessels form a rich plexus on the anterior part of the septum – Little's area or 'Keisselbachs plexus' (Fig. 21.1). This is a common site of bleeding. Bleeding is less common from the lateral nasal wall, but more difficult to control. Nosebleeds in young patients

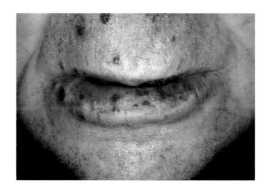

Figure 21.1 The lesions of hereditary telangiectasia.

Table 21.1 Causes of epistaxis

Local causes	General causes
Spontaneous	Cardiovascular conditions
Trauma	Hypertension, raised venous pressure
Tumours	Coagulation or vessel defects
Hereditary telangiectasia (Fig. 21.1)	Haemophilia
Nasal allergy	Leukaemia
	Anticoagulant therapy
	Thrombocytopaenia
	Fevers (rare)
	Influenza

usually settle quickly as the blood clots and the vessels go into spasm. In elderly patients the vessels are rigid and atheromatous. Nosebleeds can be persistent, serious and life-threatening.

Aetiology

Some common causes are given in Table 21.1. Most nosebleeds are idiopathic. Spontaneous epistaxis is common in children and young adults; it usually arises from Little's area or from a prominent vein just below. It may be precipitated by infection or minor trauma, is easy to stop, but tends to recur. Nosebleeds in the elderly are far more difficult to treat. The bleeding site is often high up in the posterior part of the nose and on the lateral nasal wall.

Treatment

Resuscitation and first-aid treatment

Treating active epistaxis is a very messy business – cover up your own clothes first. Now assess the patient and consider resuscitation.

Direct digital pressure on the lower nose compresses the vessel on the septum and will arrest bleeding from Little's area. Pressure over the nasal bones is useless. Examine the nose with a good light source. Gently remove clots and stale blood with suction. Now apply direct digital pressure to the nose for 10 min. The patient should sit leaning forward and breathe through the mouth. Swallowing, which may dislodge a clot, is discouraged. If bleeding persists and the site is clearly visible, e.g. Little's area, you may be able to stop it by cautery with a silver nitrate impregnated stick (Fig. 21.2). This is easier if you first put in a plug of cotton wool or ribbon gauze soaked in lidocaine and phenylephrine and leave it for 5 min. This also facilitates nasal packing but may not be practical if there is torrential bleeding.

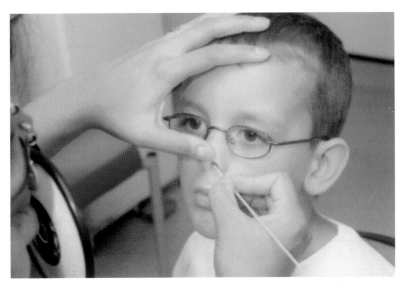

Figure 21.2 Silver nitrate stick applied to Little's area.

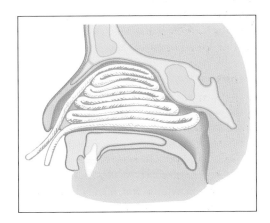

Figure 21.3 Anterior nasal packing.

Nasal packing

If simple measures fail to control the bleeding, the nose will need to be packed. One inch ribbon gauze is traditional (Fig. 21.3). The pack is introduced along the floor of the nose and built up in loops, applying even pressure to the nasal mucosa.

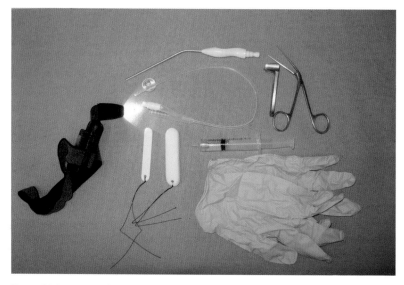

Figure 21.4 Items used to control nosebleeds.

Alternatively, one of a variety of inflatable epistaxis 'balloons' such as the 'Brighton balloon' (Fig. 21.4) can be used. It is easier to put in but may not be as effective as a well-placed pack. An easier option which causes less local trauma is to use self-expanding packs (nasal tampons) such as Merocel (Fig. 21.4) which enlarge in the presence of moisture. If bleeding continues despite adequate packing, call an ENT surgeon who may need to insert a 'post-nasal' pack. This is usually introduced under a general anaesthetic and fills the nasopharynx. A post-nasal pack is uncomfortable and causes marked airway obstruction. Patients need to be especially carefully monitored.

Patients with epistaxis severe enough to need packing should be admitted to hospital. With bed rest and sedation, most cases will settle. The blood pressure should be monitored and the haemoglobin level checked. Coexistent hypertension may need to be controlled.

Persistent bleeding

Patients can continue to bleed despite adequate packing and resuscitation. Surgery may be needed if the bleeding is from behind a cartilaginous nasal septal spur or if septal deviation prevents packing nasal septal surgery can be considered. Recalcitrant bleeds may require ligation of the ethmoidal arteries via the medial orbit, ligation of the external carotid artery or, more often nowadays, of the sphenopalatine artery by nasal endoscopic surgery.

Angiography and vessel embolization may rarely be considered.

Recurrent nosebleeds

Children are particularly susceptible to multiple nosebleeds. There may be minor inflammation of the nasal vestibule when daily application of a steroid/antibiotic cream or some petroleum jelly may help. Referral to an ENT surgeon for thorough nasal examination and cautery should be considered if simple measures fail.

Clinical practice point

• Epistaxis can kill. Particularly in elderly patients, early circulatory resuscitation, intravenous access and cross-matching may be needed before the bleed can be controlled.

Chapter 22

The nasal septum

Septal deviation

The nasal septum is rarely exactly in the midline (Fig. 22.1). Minor deviations are normal. Marked deviation will cause nasal airway obstruction. Septal deviation can be corrected by surgery, with excellent results.

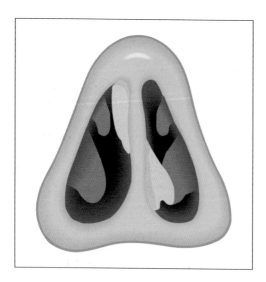

Figure 22.1 'S'-shaped deviation of the nasal septum with hypertrophy of the right middle turbinate.

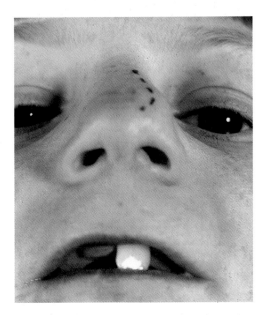

Figure 22.2 The dorsal line of the nasal septum has been marked and is displaced to the left, causing external nasal deformity in addition to nasal obstruction.

Aetiology

Most cases of deviated nasal septum (DNS) result from trauma, either recent or long forgotten, perhaps during birth. 'Buckling' in children may become more pronounced as the septum grows.

Effects

- Nasal obstruction may be unilateral or bilateral.
- Recurrent sinus infection due to impairment of sinus ventilation by the displaced septum. The middle turbinate on the concave side of the septum may hypertrophy and interfere with sinus ventilation.
- Otitis media. DNS may impair the ability to equalize middle-ear pressure, especially in divers.
- Nosebleeds – a sharp spur can be a focus for epistaxis (Fig. 22.2).

Treatment

If symptoms are minimal and only a minor degree of deviation is present, no treatment is needed. Minor septal deviations are often an incidental finding in patients with allergic rhinitis. Treat the rhinitis rather than the septal deviation.

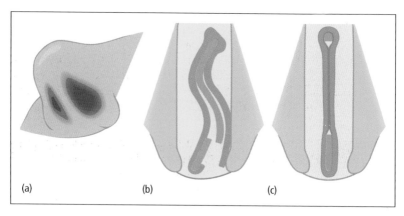

(a) (b) (c)

Figure 22.3 Nasal septal surgery (septoplasty). (a) Incision through the muco-perichondrium. (b) Elevation of muco-perichondrial flaps on either side of the septal skeleton. (c) The displaced cartilage and bone have been resected, allowing the septum to resume a midline position.

Where symptoms are more severe correction of the septal deformity is justified (though never essential).

Surgery involves elevating mucosal flaps from the septal cartilage and resecting part of the deviated cartilage before replacing it in the midline (septoplasty; Fig. 22.3). The older operation of submucous resection in which the entire septal cartilage is removed is too radical. Septal surgery should be undertaken with caution if at all in children as it may interfere with the growth of the mid-face.

Septal perforation

Aetiology

Perforation of the nasal septum may result from the following conditions:
- Nasal surgery.
- Trauma including repeated nose-picking.
- Chronic inflammation, e.g. Wegener's granulomatosis, syphilis.
- Inhalation of fumes, e.g. chrome salts.
- Cocaine.
- Carcinoma.

Effects

Many septal perforations cause no trouble. They may give rise to epistaxis and crusting or rarely whistling on inspiration or expiration. A perforation is readily seen and often has unhealthy edges covered with large crusts.

Treatment

Septal perforations are very difficult to repair.

Nasal douching with saline or bicarbonate solution reduces crusting around the edge of the defect, and antiseptic cream will control infection. If crusting and bleeding remain a problem, the perforation can be closed using a silastic double-flanged button.

Clinical practice point

- Minor deviations of the basal septum are normal. If the patient has nasal symptoms, rhinitis is a far more common cause. Treat it first.

Chapter 23

Miscellaneous nasal infections

Acute coryza

The common cold is the result of viral infection but secondary bacterial infection may supervene. It is self-limiting and no treatment is required other than an antipyretic, such as paracetamol. Discouraged the prolonged use (more than 5 days) of vasoconstrictor nose drops owing to their harmful effect on the nasal mucosa (rhinitis medicamentosa). Many patients use menthol inhalations, systemic decongestants and a variety of cough linctus preparations, and find these helpful in controlling symptoms.

Nasal vestibulitis

Both children and adults may be carriers of pyogenic staphylococci, which can produce infection of the skin of the nasal vestibule. The site becomes sore, fissured and crusted. Treatment, which needs to be prolonged, consists of topical antibiotic/antiseptic ointment. Consider systemic flucloxacillin in more severe cases. In children with persistent vestibulitis look for a nasal foreign body.

Furunculosis

An abscess in a hair follicle is rare but must be treated seriously as it can spread rapidly and lead to cavernous sinus thrombosis and meningitis. The tip of the nose becomes red, tense and painful. Give systemic antibiotics without delay, preferably by injection. Drainage may be necessary but should be deferred until the patient has had adequate antibiotic treatment for 24h. In recurrent cases, diabetes must be excluded.

Chronic purulent rhinitis

Children are especially susceptible to chronic purulent nasal discharge. The discharge is thick, mucoid, incessant and often resistant to treatment. In such cases, a nasal swab may show the presence of *Haemophilus influenzae*, which should be treated with a prolonged course of antibiotics (amoxycillin, cefaclor). In persistent cases it is important to exclude immunological deficiency, cystic fibrosis and ciliary dysfunction as well as more obvious causes, such as enlarged infected adenoids, foreign body or allergic rhinitis.

Atrophic rhinitis (ozaena)

Fortunately now uncommon in Western society, this disease is still seen occasionally. The nasal mucosa undergoes squamous metaplasia followed by atrophy, and the nose becomes filled with evil-smelling crusts. The stench is detectable even at a considerable distance. Such a patient will be ostracized and children will be shunned by their peers.

The aetiology of atrophic rhinitis is unknown. Various forms of treatment have been tried. In the early stages, meticulous attention to sinusitis and nasal hygiene may be helpful. In the more established case, the use of 50% glucose in glycerine as nasal drops seems to reduce the smell and crusting.

Various surgical measures have been devised, the most reliable of which is closure of the nostrils, using a circumferential flap of vestibular skin. After a prolonged period of closure, recovery of the nasal mucosa may occur and the nose can be reopened (Young's operation).

Clinical practice point
• Assume a child with a unilateral nasal discharge has a nasal foreign body.

Chapter 24

Acute and chronic sinusitis (rhinosinusitis)

Applied basic science

The paranasal sinuses are a series of air-filled cavities that communicate directly with the nose. They are lined with nasal mucosa and are subject to the same diseases as the nose itself – notably inflammatory processes. Hence the term 'rhinosinusitis' is more accurate than 'sinusitis'.

The *maxillary sinus* or 'antrum' is the largest of the sinuses with a capacity in the adult of approximately 15 mL. The orbit lies above and the hard palate with the roots of the second premolar and the first two molar teeth forms the floor. Medially the antrum is separated from the nose by the lateral nasal wall made up of the middle and inferior turbinate bones, each with a corresponding recess or 'meatus' below it (Fig. 24.1).

The *ethmoidal sinuses* form a honeycomb of air cells between the 'lamina papyracea' or thin bone at the medial wall of the orbit and the upper part of the nose. An upward extension forms the fronto-nasal duct draining the *frontal sinus*. The frontal sinus is within the frontal bone in the forehead and the sphenoidal sinus is in the midline within the sphenoid bone behind the nose.

The openings of the sinuses under the middle turbinate form the *ostiomeatal complex*. It is now recognized that abnormality of this area leads to failure of sinus drainage and thence to sinusitis. Abnormalities may be structural, as with a large aerated cell blocking the ostial openings. Functional anomalies such as oedema, allergy or polyp formation can also obstruct the ostiomeatal complex.

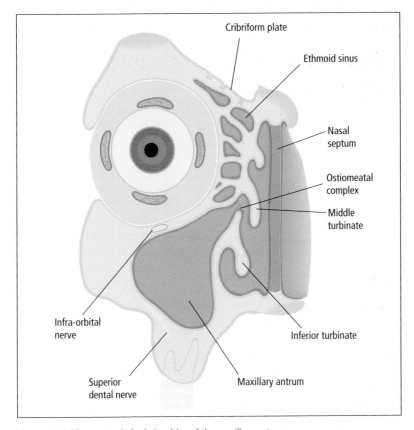

Cribriform plate

Ethmoid sinus

Nasal septum

Ostiomeatal complex

Middle turbinate

Infra-orbital nerve

Inferior turbinate

Superior dental nerve

Maxillary antrum

Figure 24.1 The anatomical relationships of the maxillary antrum.

Acute infection

Clinical features

Acute sinusitis (rhinosinusitis) is characterized by nasal discharge (rhinorhoea) and a feeling of congestion and obstruction in the nose and face. Most infections are initially viral but bacterial infection soon supervenes causing purulent rhinorhoea, increasing congestion with facial pain, nasal obstruction and in severe cases a pyrexial illness. In maxillary sinusitis the pain is mainly over the cheeks, ethmoidal and frontal sinusitis cause periorbital pain and headache, and sphenoidal sinusitis causes severe deep-seated headache. Usually more than one sinus is involved (*pan-sinusitis*; Fig. 24.2). Mucopus is apparent on inspection of the nose and there is tenderness over the involved sinuses. Beware cheek

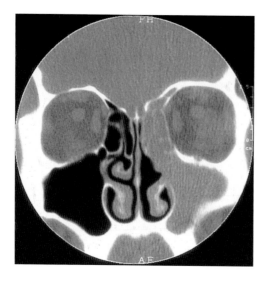

Figure 24.2 Coronal CT scan showing left-sided ethmoidal and maxillary sinusitis.

swelling, it may indicate a dental abscess. In uncomplicated sinusitis X-rays are unhelpful. The diagnosis should be made clinically.

Aetiology

Most cases of acute sinusitis are secondary to acute viral illness, e.g. coryza, which causes nasal mucosal oedema and interferes with ventilation and mucous clearance from the sinuses. The causative organisms are usually pyogenic, e.g. *Streptococcus pneumoniae*, *Haemophilus influenzae* or *Staphylococcus pyogenes*. Anaerobes may be involved in dental infections.

Many patients have a background of rhinitis, often allergic in origin, which predisposes them to episodes of ostiomeatal complex obstruction and sinus infection.

In about 10% of cases of maxillary sinusitis the infection is dental in origin and has spread from the upper molars or premolars. Occasionally, infection follows the entry of infected material, e.g. after diving – water is forced through the ostium, into the sinus.

Treatment

- Adequate analgesia.
- If the nasal discharge is mucopurulent, give antibiotics. Cefaclor is a useful first-line.

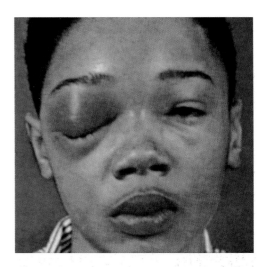

Figure 24.3 Orbital cellulitis.

• Vasoconstrictor nose drops, such as 1% ephedrine or 0.05% oxymetazoline, will aid drainage of the sinus. Use these sparingly and only for short periods (3–5 days is enough).

Acute sinusitis usually resolves without complications. If the ostiomeatal complex is completely obstructed there may be severe pain due to retained pus (empyaema). If so the now rarely performed 'antral washout' – insertion of a trochar into the antrum via the nasal cavity with aspiration of the contents of the antrum – will bring about dramatic relief.

Complications of acute rhinosinusitis

Complications may arise if the infection spreads beyond the bony walls of the sinuses (Fig. 24.3). These are rare in Western communities but still a significant cause of morbidity and mortality worldwide. Beware of the patient with sinusitis who develops severe headache, swinging pyrexia or neurological signs:

• Orbital complications (cellulitis or abscess) are characterized by marked oedema of the eyelids, diplopia, redness and swelling of the conjunctiva (chemosis). Proptosis indicates severe orbital involvement. Commence intravenous antibiotics immediately and ask for an urgent ENT opinion. Resolution usually follows intensive antibiotic therapy but surgical drainage is required urgently if there is any change in vision. Loss of colour discrimination is an early sign of impending visual loss.

• Meningitis, extradural and subdural abscesses may occur and should be treated as neurosurgical emergencies.

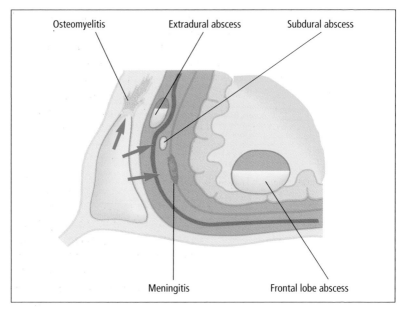

Figure 24.4 Complications of frontal sinusitis.

• Cerebral abscess (frontal lobe) deserves special mention in view of the insidious nature of its development. Any patient who has a history of recent frontal sinus infection and complains of headaches, is apathetic or exhibits any abnormality of behaviour should be suspected of harbouring a frontal lobe abscess.

• Osteomyelitis of the frontal bone is characterized by persistent headache and oedema of the scalp in the vicinity of the frontal sinus. X-ray signs are late, and by the time they become apparent osteomyelitis is well established. Intensive antibiotic therapy combined with removal of diseased bone is necessary.

• Cavernous sinus thrombosis is very rare. Proptosis, chemosis and ophthalmoplegia characterize this dangerous complication (Fig. 24.4).

Recurrent and chronic infection

Many patients suffer repeated misery due to frequent and recurrent episodes of rhinosinusitis. Referral to an ENT surgeon is important so that anatomical abnormalities, e.g. nasal septal deviations, ostiomeatal complex anomalies, and ciliary and immunological function can be checked for. The patient may have nasal polyposis or allergic rhinitis. Acute sinusitis may fail to resolve and the patient goes on to complain of constant nasal discharge, congestion and facial pain.

Anosmia (loss of smell) and nasal obstruction are common. Examination will show an inflamed nasal mucosa and mucopurulent discharge. In many patients there is an active allergic rhinitis and this must be controlled before any surgery is considered. Treatment is by systemic antibiotics – often for prolonged periods – and topical intranasal steroids. Intranasal steroids are a good first-line treatment for any form of chronic rhinitis. A therapeutic trial of nasal steroids can be given before referral to an ENT surgeon. Symptomatic treatment may involve nasal douches with saline, and judicious occasional use of nasal decongestants.

Surgery (functional endoscopic sinus surgery)

If surgery is considered necessary, it is now usual to establish drainage of the sinuses by endoscopic surgery of the ostiomeatal area under the middle turbinate – functional endoscopic sinus surgery (FESS). Developments in endoscopic instruments now allow inspection of the sinus ostia and interior of the paranasal sinuses. Ostial enlargement and removal of polyps and cysts can be performed. The ostiomeatal complex under the middle turbinate is opened up. This allows a more 'physiological' drainage of the antrum than was possible before the development of endoscopic endonasal surgery.

Clinical practice point

• Most cases of sinusitis resolve but complications can be devastating. Beware of the sinusitis patient with severe headache, suspected neurological signs or orbital swelling.

Chapter 25

Tumours of the nose, sinuses and nasopharynx

These tumours are rare and often not diagnosed until they have spread to surrounding structures.

Carcinoma of the maxillary antrum (Fig. 25.1)

Clinical features

In its earliest stages it will give rise to no symptoms. Blood-stained nasal discharge and increasing unilateral nasal obstruction should raise suspicion. One of the risk factors for development of adenocarcinoma of the maxillary antrum is exposure to the resins produced by hardwoods and it is important to take a careful occupational history.

Late features are sadly often the presenting features and include:

- Swelling of the cheek.
- Swelling or ulceration of the gums or palate.
- Epiphora, owing to involvement of the nasolacrimal duct.
- Proptosis and diplopia, due to involvement of the floor of the orbit.
- Pain – commonly in the cheek, but may be referred to the ear, head or jaw.

Lymphatic spread is to the submandibular and deep cervical nodes and occurs late.

Treatment

The tumour may be too far advanced for curative treatment at presentation. A combination of surgery and radiotherapy offers the best chance. Total maxillectomy (with exenteration of the orbit if involved) may be needed. This results

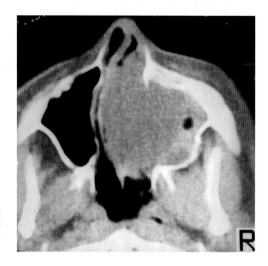

Figure 25.1 CT scan showing large carcinoma of the right maxillary antrum with extension into the right nasal cavity.

in fenestration of the hard palate, for which a modified upper denture with an obturator is provided. The fenestration allows drainage and access for inspection of the antral cavity. Following maxillectomy, a radical course of radiotherapy is given.

Even with radical treatment, carcinoma of the antrum has a poor prognosis, with only about 30% of patients surviving to 5 years.

Carcinoma of the ethmoid sinuses

The clinical features are similar to those of maxillary carcinoma, but invasion of the orbit and facial skin below the inner canthus is early. Treatment is by radical surgery and radiotherapy.

Malignant disease of the nasopharynx

This is rare in Europe but relatively common in the Far East in general and in southern China in particular.

Aetiology

The Epstein–Barr virus may play a role in the aetiology of nasopharyngeal malignancy. Dietary factors may partly explain the increased risk in South China. Virtually all malignant tumours of the nasopharynx are squamous cell carcinomas – rarely lymphoma or adenoid cystic carcinoma.

Clinical features

There may be no initial local symptoms:
- Nasal obstruction and blood-stained nasal discharge are usually late.
- Unilateral otitis media with effusion is thought to result from Eustachian tube obstruction. Patients may present with conductive deafness. Maintain a high index of suspicion, especially in Chinese patients.
- Invasion of the skull base causes involvement of various cranial nerves, especially nerves V (paraesthesia in the face and corneal anaesthesia), VI (ophthalmoplegia), IX (pain in the throat, loss of gag reflex), X (hoarseness) and XII (abnormal tongue movement).
- Spread to the upper deep cervical nodes occurs early and may be bilateral. Such a node is typically wedged between the mastoid process and angle of the jaw.

Treatment

Treatment of nasopharyngeal cancer is by radiotherapy following confirmatory biopsy. Once the primary site has been controlled, radical neck dissection is carried out if there were involved nodes at diagnosis or if any subsequently develop. The prognosis is poor, but the earlier the diagnosis is made, the better the outlook.

Other tumours of the nasal region

Osteomata

Osteomata are benign bony tumours usually in the frontal and ethmoidal sinuses. They are slow-growing and cause few symptoms but may eventually call for surgical removal.

Nasopharyngeal angiofibroma

Nasopharyngeal angiofibroma is a rare benign tumour of adolescent boys. It presents as epistaxis and nasal obstruction, and is usually easily visible by posterior rhinoscopy. Being highly vascular, the tumour is locally destructive and extends into the surrounding structures. Diagnosis is confirmed by MR scanning and treatment is by surgical removal.

Malignant granuloma

Though not truly neoplastic, malignant granuloma is a sinister condition characterized by progressive ulceration of the nose and neighbouring structures. This is probably a variant of lymphoma.

Malignant melanoma

Malignant melanoma is fortunately rare in the nose and sinuses. Treatment is by radical surgery but the prognosis is extremely poor.

Clinical practice points

- Paranasal sinus and post-nasal space tumours present late.
- The combination of unilateral deafness, enlarged cervical nodes and cranial nerve palsies must be considered to be due to nasopharyngeal cancer.

Chapter 26

Rhinitis and nasal polyps

Rhinitis

The misery brought about by inflammation of the nose is one of the commonest reasons for patients to consult a GP or ENT surgeon. Many patients self-medicate, miss time from work or school, and may develop severe asthma as part of a general pattern of respiratory tract allergy.

Applied basic science

The nasal mucosa is at the entrance of the respiratory tract. It is made up of ciliated epithelium and produces a mucus blanket which helps protect the airway from inspired pollutants, allergens and infective agents. The epithelium is continuous with that of the rest of the respiratory system and is subject to much the same pathologies. Inflammation of the nasal mucosa (rhinitis) is common and in one form or another affects everyone at some time. Rhinitis is caused primarily by allergy or infection (Chapter 24, Acute and Chronic Sinusitis 'Rhinosinusitis').

Allergic rhinitis is on the increase. In developed Western societies as many as one child in four has some degree of nasal allergy. The main allergens are pollens, particularly troublesome in the spring and early summer (seasonal allergic rhinitis or 'hay fever'), the ubiquitous house-dust mite which lives on desquamated human skin (Fig. 26.1), animal dander (e.g. from cats or dogs) and, less often, mould spores which are particularly active in autumn. The allergen induces production of IgE antibodies which on subsequent exposure bind with the allergen to form antigen-antibody complexes. These complexes then attach

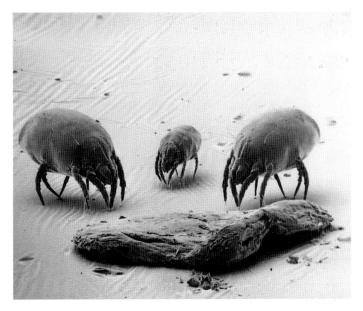

Figure 26.1 Scanning electron micrograph of house-dust mites and a human squame. (Crown copyright reproduced by kind permission of Dr D.A. Griffiths, Head of Storage Pests Department, Slough Laboratory, London Road, Slough.)

to mast cells in the nasal epithelium, causing the cells to rupture and release inflammatory mediators including histamine. (Type 1 allergic response, Fig. 26.2(a) and (b).) An intense local inflammatory reaction ensues with oedema and secretion of mucus. The nose may now become sensitive to irritants in inspired air, so that the slightest stimulus will cause symptoms to recur.

Clinical features

The main symptoms are:
- nasal congestion
- nasal obstruction
- rhinorrhoea or a watery nasal discharge
- sneezing
- reduced or absent sense of smell (hyposmia or anosmia).

Take a careful history and enquire particularly about other manifestations of allergy, e.g. eczema and asthma. The association with asthma is very strong – many patients will have both allergic rhinitis and asthma. 'Atopy' or a

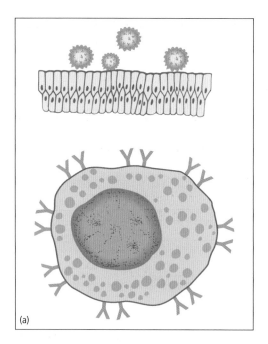

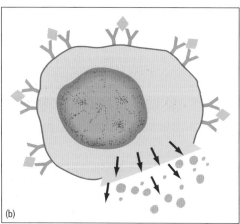

Figure 26.2 (a) A mast cell showing intracellular granules and antibodies attached to the cell wall. (b) Further exposure to antigen has resulted in rupture of the cell wall and release of the mast cell granules.

predisposition to develop allergies is often inherited and there may be a strong family history.

Signs are few, but examine the nose and look for redness or swelling of the mucosa – particularly the turbinates – and a mucoid discharge. Check for structural anomalies such a septal deviation or nasal polyps, but even if these are noted it is wise to treat the rhinitis. Investigations are not usually needed but sensitivity tests for specific allergens – 'skin prick tests' – may help to direct allergen avoidance therapy.

Treatment

- Allergen avoidance measures include minimizing contact with house-dust or pollens.
- Systemic or intranasal antihistamines help control symptoms.
- Intranasal steroids – the mainstay of treatment.
- Sodium chromoglycate – stabilizes mast cells.
- Nasal decongestants – use sparingly and briefly if at all.
- Leukotriene receptor antagonists – currently undergoing trials.

Other forms of 'rhinitis'

Atrophic rhinitis is covered in Chapter 23.

Hormonal rhinitis

Puberty, pregnancy and the menopause are occasions of greatly changed hormonal activity and some degree of nasal congestion, rhinorhoea and sneezing may occur at these times.

Senile rhinitis

Elderly patients may develop troublesome rhinorhoea, causing a 'drip' at the end of the nose. This often responds well to ipratroprium bromide, an atropine-like spray.

'Vasomotor' rhinitis

Variation in the state of engorgement of the nasal mucosa is normal (Fig. 26.3) – the nasal cycle. For some patients, this causes troublesome nasal obstruction and the term 'vasomotor rhinitis' is used. A trial of intranasal steroids may be helpful. These patients should be discouraged from repeated use of nasal decongestants due to the risk of rhinitis medicamentosa.

Rhinitis medicamentosa

Excessive use of nasal decongestants causes rebound nasal congestion. Treatment is to stop the drops or sprays.

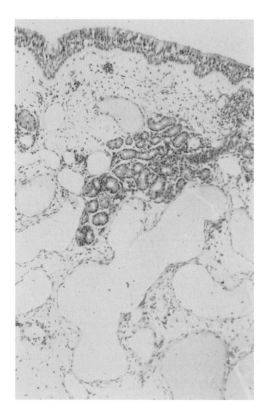

Figure 26.3 View of nasal turbinate mucosa showing the many blood vessels within the substance. (Slide courtesy of Dr Roger Start.)

Cerebrospinal fluid leak

Very rarely an apparent mucoid secretion from the nose is cerebrospinal fluid (CSF) which has leaked from the brain. This typically occurs after head injury or as a complication of nasal surgery.

Nasal polyps

Nasal polyps are composed of swollen and oedematous nasal mucosal tissues. They can cause complete nasal obstruction.

Polyps are yellowish-grey, smooth and moist (Fig. 26.4). They are pedunculated and move on gentle probing although they are insensitive, unlike the inferior turbinate. It is common to see the inferior turbinate and mistake it for a polyp – do not be caught out.

Nasal polyps may be a feature of long-standing rhinitis of any cause. They are thought to arise mainly from the mucosa of the ethmoid sinuses which

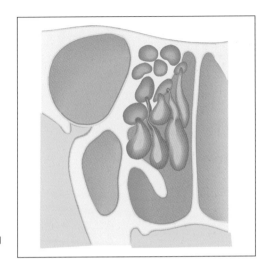

Figure 26.4 Multiple ethmoidal polyps.

gradually swells until it projects into the nose, giving the polyps a pedunculated appearance. Histologically, nasal polyps consist of a loose oedematous stroma infiltrated by inflammatory lymphocytes and eosinophils and covered by respiratory epithelium.

Beware of nasal polyps in children. Think of cystic fibrosis or in a newborn baby a nasal glioma or a nasal encephalocele.

Treatment

Topical steroids may be adequate for small polyps.
A short course of systemic steroids is useful in severe cases.

Nasal polypectomy involves avulsion of the polyps or removal by powered micro-resector, usually combined with endoscopic clearance of the ethmoid sinuses (FESS, see Chapter 24).

Unilateral nasal polyps

Nasal polyposis is usually a mucosal disease and presents in both the nostrils. Beware of unilateral polyps, which may represent a neoplastic lesion. More often, a unilateral polyp is an 'antrochoanal' polyp. This is usually solitary and benign, arising within the maxillary antrum, extruding through the ostium and presenting as a smooth swelling in the nasopharynx (Fig. 26.5). Such a polyp may extend below the soft palate and be several centimetres in length. Treatment is surgical removal.

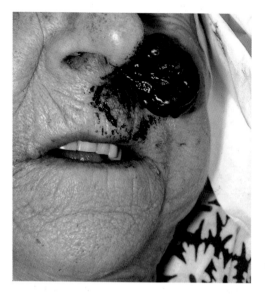

Figure 26.5 A nasal polyp which has prolapsed out of the nose.

Clinical practice points

- An intranasal steroid is a good first-line treatment for rhinitis of any cause.
- Beware of unilateral nasal polyps and polyps in children.

Chapter 27

Choanal atresia

The posterior nasal apertures or 'choanae' may fail to canalize in the growing embryo. The primitive membrane – bucconasal membrane – which separates the nose from the nasopharynx then persists causing nasal obstruction in the newborn baby. This condition is fortunately rare –1 in 8000 live births. It is often accompanied by other congenital anomalies. The acronym 'CHARGE' refers to the various anomalies that are often clustered together – Colobomata (an anomaly of the eye), Heart anomalies, Atresia of the choanae, Renal anomalies, Genital hypoplasia, Ear deformity.

Bilateral atresia

This is a life-threatening condition presenting in the newborn baby with airway obstruction. The airway obstruction is relieved by crying. Without immediate first-aid treatment with an oral airway the baby will asphyxiate. Such an airway should be fixed in place with tape, and the diagnosis is confirmed by the inability to pass a catheter through the nose into the pharynx. A useful test is to place a cold steel tongue depressor under the baby's nostrils and look for misting (Chapter 18). CT scanning shows the atresia clearly (Fig. 27.1).

Treatment

Treatment is by surgery performed by the transnasal route under endoscopic control.

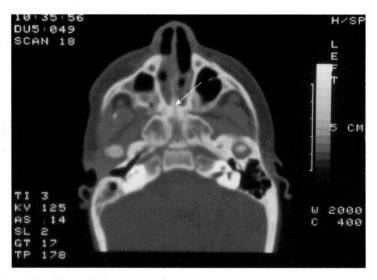

Figure 27.1 CT scan of bilateral choanal atresia.

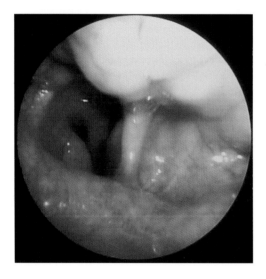

Figure 27.2 Endoscopic view of unilateral congenital posterior choanal atresia. The atretic plate can be clearly seen, and on the patent side the posterior ends of the inferior and middle turbinates are visible.

Unilateral atresia

The condition may pass unrecognized until the age of 5–10 years when it becomes apparent that one nostril is occluded and thick mucus accumulates. Testing with a probe and examination by posterior rhinoscopy will confirm the diagnosis (Fig. 27.2).

Treatment

Correction of choanal atresia is performed transnasally, usually with a drill, while observing the choana from the postnasal aspect with a 120° telescope.

Clinical practice point

- Bilateral choanal atresia is a life-threatening emergency. Secure an oral airway and refer to ENT immediately.

Chapter 28

Adenoids

Applied basic science

The adenoids are part of a circle of lymphoid tissue – *Waldeyer's ring* – which surrounds the entrance to the upper aerodigestive tract (UAT). Waldeyer's ring includes the palatine tonsils, lymphoid tissue in the tongue base – lingual tonsils – and a few discrete aggregates of submucosal lymphoid follicles dispersed throughout the pharynx. The adenoids are found in the nasopharynx, behind the soft palate projecting from the posterior pharyngeal wall. They occupy a large part of the space in the nasopharynx in young children. Their function is that of the pharyngeal lymphoid tissue in general, i.e. to mount an immunological response to infective agents. They are small at birth, enlarge due to hypertrophy and hyperplasia during the first 5 years of life, and regress from about the age of 7 years to adolescence, when they have all but disappeared.

In some children – mainly up to the age of 5 years – repeated upper respiratory infections cause pathological adenoidal enlargement so that the airway is obstructed. The child will mouth-breathe, snore continuously and in severe cases develop obstructive sleep apnoea (OSA) – Chapter 30. Continued mouth breathing causes drying of the throat and predisposes to chest infections. The submucosal lymphoid tissue is colonized by bacteria and may give rise to repeated upper respiratory infections, in particular rhinosinusitis and otitis media. It is thought that bacteria in the adenoids can form a protective polymeric matrix (**biofilm**) which makes penetration by antibiotics and the child's host defence mechanisms difficult. The sheer bulk of the adenoids may obstruct the opening of the Eustachian tube and contribute to middle ear disease in this way. 'Adenoidal' children may have a hyponasal quality to their speech as the normal resonance associated with a clear nasopharynx is lost, e.g. the child will pronounce '*mummy and nanny*' as '*bubby and daddy*'.

Adenoids are often incorrectly blamed for a variety of childhood conditions. The main adverse effects of adenoids are:

- nasal obstruction
- pharyngitis (due to dry mouth)
- obstructive sleep apnoea
- rhinosinusitis
- recurrent upper respiratory infections
- otitis media.

Presentation and diagnosis

The history will confirm the features mentioned above. Nasal obstruction and mouth breathing are often apparent during the consultation. The adenoids are not seen during a routine examination of the nose and throat but a good view can now be had with an endoscope introduced into the nose, a procedure often surprisingly well tolerated by children (Fig. 28.1). Enlarged adenoids can also be seen by mirror examination (Fig. 28.2). A lateral soft tissue X-ray of the neck will show a shadow in the postnasal space delineating the adenoids (Fig. 28.3).

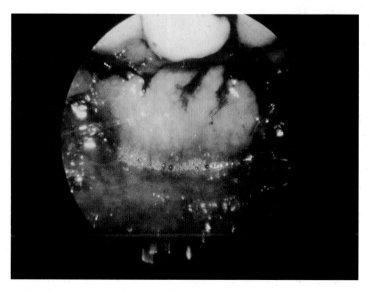

Figure 28.1 Endoscopic view of the adenoids.

117

Treatment

Adenoidectomy is considered for rhinitis that fails to respond to medical treatment, in OSA and in some cases of otitis media, particularly otitis media with effusion (OME, Chapter 12) that has recurred despite previous treatment with grommets. In children with recurrent ear disease, there is some evidence that 'adjuvant adenoidectomy' i.e. adenoidectomy in conjunction with grommet insertion improves outcomes in younger children.

Adenoidectomy is carried out under general anaesthesia with endotracheal intubation. An adenoid curette is swept down the posterior pharyngeal wall,

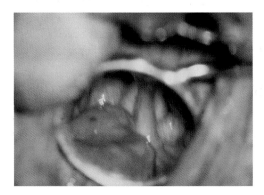

Figure 28.2 Mirror view of the nasopharynx showing adenoid tissue and the posterior end of the nasal septum (viewed under general anaesthetic).

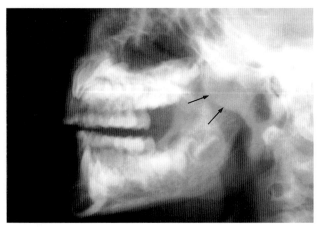

Figure 28.3 A lateral soft tissue X-ray showing adenoid enlargement.

taking care to remove all remnants of lymphoid tissues. Some ENT surgeons prefer to use a suction-diathermy device under direct vision to reduce bleeding.

Complications

- Haemorrhage – this usually occurs in the first 24 hours. Do not delay in setting up a drip, getting blood cross-matched and returning the child to theatre. *Delay may be fatal*. A postnasal pack is inserted under general anaesthetic after first making sure that there are no tags of adenoid tissues left.
- Otitis media.
- Regrowth of residual adenoid tissue.
- *'Rhinolalia aperta'*. This is a disorder of speech characterized by escape of air from the nose during articulation. Removal of large adenoids in a child with a short soft palate may result in palatal incompetence. Resolution usually occurs without treatment, but if not, speech therapy is advisable.

Clinical practice points

- The indications for adenoidectomy are often very different to the indications for tonsillectomy.
- Assess each child for adenoidectomy on an individual basis rather than automatically suggesting 'adenotonsillectomy'.

Chapter 29

The oropharynx and tonsils

Applied basic science

The pharynx is divided into three parts – the nasopharynx (post-nasal space) between the skull base and the hard palate, the oropharynx between the hard palate and the hyoid bone, and the hypopharynx between the hyoid bone and the lower part of the cricoid cartilage of the larynx (Fig. 29.1).

The tonsils are in the oropharynx.

Acute and chronic pharyngitis

Acute pharyngitis is common and probably starts as a virus infection. It is often associated with acute rhinosinusitis as part of an upper respiratory infection.

The patient complains of dysphagia and malaise; on examination, the mucosa is hyperaemic.

Chronic pharyngitis produces a persistent though mild soreness of the throat, usually with a complaint of dryness.

Predisposing factors that should be looked for are:

- Smoking (including passive smoking).
- Mouth breathing as a result of nasal obstruction.
- Rhinosinusitis.
- Periodontal disease.

Treatment is symptomatic but the causes listed above may warrant treatment in their own right.

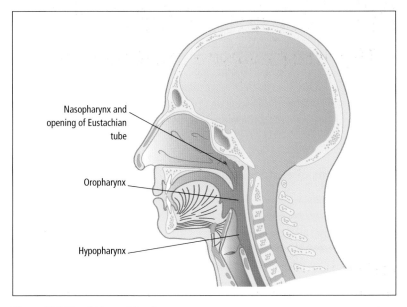

Nasopharynx and opening of Eustachian tube

Oropharynx

Hypopharynx

Figure 29.1 The divisions of the pharynx.

Acute tonsillitis

Mostly occurs in children and young adults. Initial infection is typically viral but *Streptococcus pyogenes* is an important pathogen.

Symptoms

- Sore throat and dysphagia. Swallowing is painful. Young children may not complain of sore throat but will refuse to eat.
- Earache as a result of referred pain.
- Headache and malaise.

Signs

- Pyrexia may lead to febrile convulsions in susceptible infants.
- The tonsils are enlarged and hyperaemic and may exude pus.
- The pharynx is inflamed.
- Foetor (bad breath).
- The cervical lymph nodes are enlarged and tender.

Treatment

- Paracetamol.
- Encourage the patient to drink to prevent dehydration.
- Antibiotics in severe cases. Simple viral sore throats do not warrant antibiotics which are in any case ineffective. If there is evidence of bacterial infection – e.g. pus, severe pain on swallowing or a prolonged course, penicillin remains the treatment of choice. If the child cannot swallow, intravenous antibiotics may be needed.

Complications of acute tonsillitis

- Acute otitis media.
- Peritonsillar abscess (quinsy).
- Parapharyngeal abscess.
- Retropharyngeal abscess.
- Pulmonary infections (pneumonia, etc.).
- Glomerulonephritis.
- Rheumatic fever.
- Scarlet fever.

Scarlet fever is a streptococcal tonsillitis with a punctate erythematous rash, and a 'strawberry' tongue. Rheumatic fever and glomerulonephritis are due to immune complex deposition secondary to streptococcal tonsillitis. They are now rare conditions in the developed world.

Quinsy (peritonsillar abscess)

A quinsy is a collection of pus forming outside the capsule of the tonsil. It is more common in adults than in children.

The patient, already suffering from acute tonsillitis becomes more ill, has a peak of temperature and develops severe dysphagia with referred otalgia. On examination, a most striking and constant feature is trismus; the buccal mucosa is furred and there is foetor.

The quinsy pushes the tonsil downwards and medially.

Treatment

Treatment is intravenous antibiotics and drainage of the abscess. The patient will then spit out pus and some blood, and the relief is immediate and dramatic. In children, drainage of a quinsy is rarely needed and may require general anaesthesia.

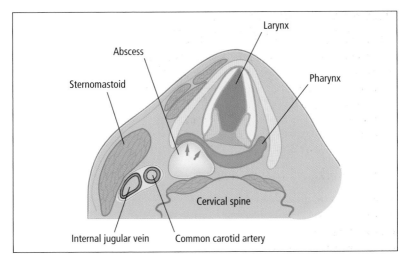

Figure 29.2 Retropharyngeal abscess. Note the proximity to the larynx and to the great vessels in the parapharyngeal space.

Retropharyngeal abscess

Infection can track in to the lymph nodes behind the pharyngeal wall especially in infants (Fig. 29.2). The child is obviously ill, dribbling and has a high temperature. There may be airway obstruction. Inspection and palpation of the posterior pharyngeal wall reveals a smooth bulge, usually on one side of the midline.

Antibiotics should be given in full doses. The child should be referred for incision of the abscess without delay. General anaesthesia is advisable but requires great skill.

Parapharyngeal abscess

Infection can spread beyond the pharynx and into the neck (Fig. 29.3). High-dose intravenous antibiotics and sometimes drainage will be needed.

Rarer forms of acute tonsillitis

Infectious mononucleosis

Infectious mononucleosis (glandular fever) usually presents as severe membranous tonsillitis. The node enlargement is marked and malaise is more severe than

123

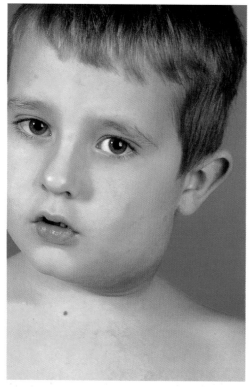

Figure 29.3 Parapharyngeal abscess.

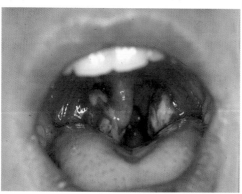

Figure 29.4 The appearance of the tonsils in glandular fever.

expected from tonsillitis (Fig. 29.4). Diagnosis is confirmed by lymphocytosis on the blood film. Within a week the *Monospot* blood test becomes positive. The cause is the Epstein–Barr virus and spread is by close contact. Adolescents are especially susceptible ('kissing disease').

Diphtheria

Diphtheria is now very rare but may still occur. It is of insidious onset and characterized by a grey membrane (difficult to remove) on the tonsils, fauces and uvula. Pyrexia is usually low and diagnosis is confirmed by examination and culture of a swab.

Agranulocytosis

Agranulocytosis is manifested by ulceration and membrane formation on the tonsils and oral mucosa. The neutropenia is diagnostic.

HIV

Patients with impaired immunity from HIV infection are particularly at risk of pharyngitis and ulcerative tonsillitis.

Recurrent acute tonsillitis

Most people will at some time experience acute tonsillitis; some are subject to recurrent attacks, especially in childhood. Between attacks the patient is usually symptom-free and the tonsils appear healthy. If such attacks are frequent and severe, tonsillectomy may be considered. The indications for tonsillectomy have changed greatly in recent years despite continuing uncertainty. The SIGN (Scottish Intercollegiate Guidance Network) guidelines are based on a review of current evidence and suggest that patients should meet all the following criteria:
- Sore throats are due to tonsillitis (check the signs and symptoms above).
- Five or more episodes of sore throat per year.
- Symptoms for at least a year.
- The episodes of sore throat are disabling and prevent normal functioning.

Tonsillectomy

Tonsillectomy rates vary greatly, not only between countries but in different regions in the same country. Tonsillectomy is undertaken in children much more frequently than in adults (2 to 1). The operation is widely performed in well-to-do Western communities, less frequently in the developing world. Indications remain controversial, but the evidence base is improving. Common reasons for tonsillectomy are:
- Recurrent sore throats (see SIGN guidelines above).
- Obstructive sleep apnoea (OSA) (See Chapter 30).
- Suspected malignancy or lymphoma.

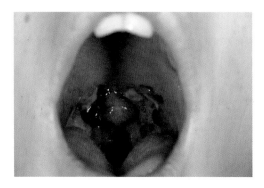

Figure 29.5 The throat one day after a tonsillectomy. This appearance is normal.

Post-operative care

Tonsillectomy is painful, especially in the first 10 days or so after surgery. Adequate analgesia and hydration is essential. The appearance of the tonsil beds often causes alarm. They may be covered with a white or yellowish exudate, which persists for up 2 weeks. This is quite normal and does not indicate infection. It is not pus (Fig. 29.5).

The main complication is bleeding. This can occur at or just after surgery (**primary bleed**, sometimes needing a second operation to control the bleeding). More often it occurs in the week or so after surgery (**secondary bleed**) when it is thought to be due to infection of the tonsil beds and usually improves after a few days antibiotics.

Tonsillar enlargement

Many parents are concerned about the size of their child's tonsils but no treatment is needed unless the child is subject to recurring attacks of acute tonsillitis or the tonsils are obstructing the airway (see Chapter 30). Very rarely a lymphoma presents as a unilateral tonsillar enlargement but some degree of asymmetry of the tonsils is normal in children.

Malignant disease of the tonsil and pharynx

Carcinoma

Carcinoma will present as painful ulceration with induration of the tonsil or pharyngeal wall. There is often earache (referred pain) and slight bleeding. Lymphatic spread to the neck nodes is early.

Lymphoma

Lymphoma of the tonsil tends not to ulcerate, but produces painless enlargement of the affected tonsil.

Clinical practice points

- Most sore throats are viral, short-lived and do not require antibiotics.
- Tonsillectomy is painful. Patients need prolonged analgesia and hydration.

Chapter 30

Snoring and obstructive sleep apnoea

Snoring is the low-pitched noise brought about mainly by vibration of the pharynx during partial airway obstruction. This obstruction is typically worse when the patient is asleep because the pharyngeal muscles relax and become atonic. Snoring is a common clinical problem. The far more serious condition of **obstructive sleep apnoea (OSA)** is characterized by episodes of cessation of airflow (apnoea) during sleep despite continuing respiratory efforts (obstruction).

Predisposing factors

The predisposing factors are:
- obesity,
- conditions which cause nasal or pharyngeal obstruction e.g. rhinitis, large tonsils and adenoids in children,
- increasing age,
- alcohol,
- smoking.

Adverse effects

Snoring causes a lot of marital disharmony and social isolation. We now realize that it is part of the spectrum of sleep-related breathing disorders with OSA at the severe end. The apnoeic episodes are characterized by hypoxaemia i.e. brief reductions in blood oxygenation. This causes repeated arousals, i.e. the patient wakes himself up, and good-quality sleep is impossible. Hence these patients are tired and sleepy during the day which can affect work performance and contribute to road traffic accidents (excessive daytime sleepiness, EDS). If hypoxaemias are prolonged and repeated, this can predispose to hypertension, stroke and right-sided heart failure.

Diagnosis

Take a careful history in all patients who snore. Enquire especially about daytime sleepiness. The sleeping partner may be able to tell you if the patient stops breathing. Examine the upper respiratory tract for any evidence of obstruction and pay particular attention to the patient's weight and cardiovascular status. If there is any suspicion of OSA refer for sleep studies. These involve measuring blood oxygen tension and a variety of respiratory variable over a few hours of sleep.

Treatment

- Simple measures such as weight loss and avoidance of alcohol at night should be tried first.
- Treat rhinitis.
- For uncomplicated snoring various devices that improve the calibre of the nasal airway or splint the jaw forward to improve the pharyngeal airway in this way are available.
- For established OSA, treatment with continuous pressure inspired air delivered by a face-mask or nasal prongs at night may be needed – continuous positive airway pressure (CPAP).
- Surgery to improve the airway is a last resort and results are uncertain.

Snoring and OSA in children

Snoring is very common in the preschool child. In otherwise healthy children, it is often associated with large tonsils and adenoids. Mild snoring on its own probably needs no treatment. OSA in children can cause not daytime sleepiness but excessive activity and behaviour problems. There is increasing evidence that it can adversely affect school performance. If the child has evidence of OSA refer to an ENT surgeon who may recommend adenotonsillectomy. Snoring and OSA in children with special needs e.g. Down syndrome or cerebral palsy, can be particularly difficult to manage and referral is best.

Clinical practice point

- Snoring is not just a nuisance; it can be a serious medical problem.

Chapter 31

The larynx: applied basic science and examination

Anatomy of the larynx

The larynx or voice-box is part of the upper respiratory tract. It is lined with cili-ated columnar epithelium except over the vocal folds or 'cords' which are covered with squamous epithelium. It is made of a series of cartilages, the main ones being the epiglottis, the cricoid cartilage (a complete ring just above the trachea) and the thyroid cartilage, which is felt as the 'Adam's Apple' externally in the neck. Various membranes, muscles and ligaments complete the structure of the larynx (Figs 31.1 and 31.2).

Physiology of the larynx

Air passes through the vocal folds, which vibrate like the reed of a musical instru-ment in expiration to produce voice (phonation). The other functions of the larynx are as a conduit for air entry into the respiratory tract and to close off the air-passages during swallowing to protect the lungs.

Symptoms and signs of laryngeal disease

Lesions on or around the vocal cords cause **hoarseness**. Failure of the laryngeal inlet to close on swallowing causes **aspiration**; the patient will cough and splut-ter on swallowing. The most dangerous laryngeal pathology is narrowing of the airway. This causes reduced air entry and turbulent flow so that the patient makes a high-pitched noise when breathing (**stridor**). Increasing difficulty causes a rise in respiratory rate (tachypnoea), and the patient will struggle to breathe as

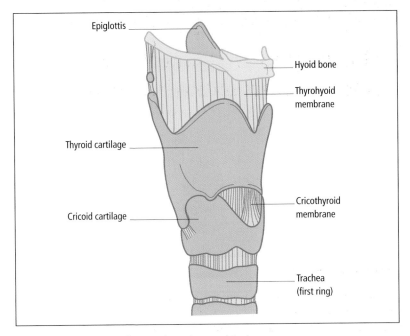

Figure 31.1 The main cartilages and membranes of the larynx.

he uses the accessory muscles of respiration to maintain airflow. In severe cases there may be cyanosis, cessation of airflow (apnoea) and death.

Examination of the larynx

You can get some idea of how the larynx is working by listening to the patient's voice (is he hoarse?) and observing his breathing (is there stridor?). It is useful to palpate the neck as well and feel for the prominence of the laryngeal cartilages. 'Crepitus' or a sensation of 'crackling' under your fingers when you gently move the larynx is normal.

Inspecting the larynx requires some skill and practice. For **indirect laryngoscopy** ask the patient to protrude his tongue, which is held gently between the examiner's middle finger and thumb (Figs 31.3 and 31.4). A warmed laryngeal mirror is introduced gently but firmly against the soft palate in the midline. By tilting the laryngeal mirror, the various structures shown in Fig. 31.2 can be seen. To assess mobility of the cords ask the patient to say 'EE', causing adduction (movement of the cords towards the midline) or to take a deep breath, which causes abduction (movement of the cords away from the midline).

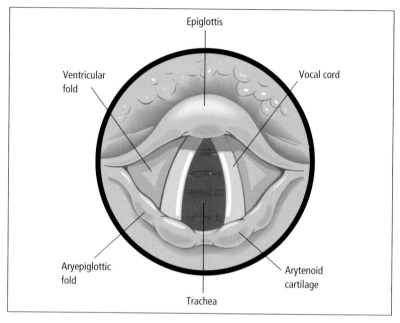

Figure 31.2 The structures seen on indirect laryngoscopy.

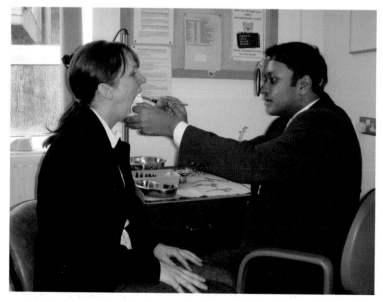

Figure 31.3 The technique of indirect laryngoscopy.

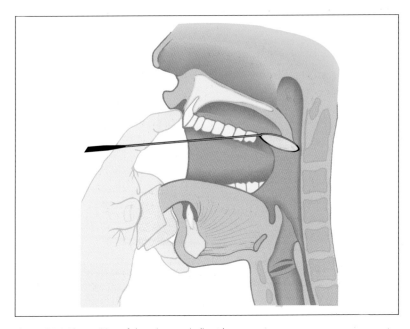

Figure 31.4 The position of the mirror on indirect laryngoscopy.

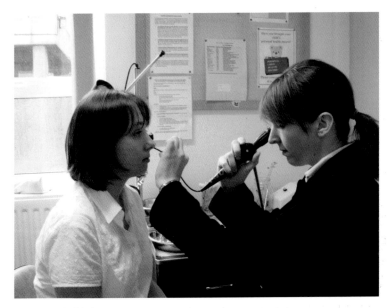

Figure 31.5 Flexible laryngoscopy.

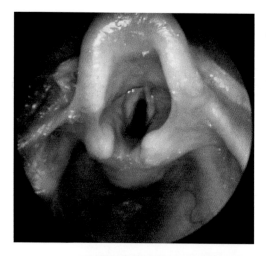

Figure 31.6 The normal larynx as seen by direct laryngoscopy in a child.

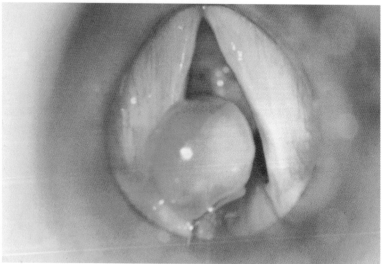

Figure 31.7 The appearance of the larynx as seen by direct laryngoscopy. Note the large polyp on the left vocal cord.

Fibre-optic laryngoscopy is increasingly available and fibre-optic instruments are now of extremely high quality. The instrument is passed through the nose into the pharynx. It is then manoeuvred past the epiglottis until the interior of the larynx is seen (Fig. 31.5). This allows inspection of the cords during phonation and also enables a photographic record to be made. The patient can even see his own larynx on a television monitor.

For more detailed examination and particularly if a biopsy is needed **direct laryngoscopy** under general anaesthesia is required (Figs 31.6 and 31.7).

Clinical practice point
• The main symptoms and signs of laryngeal disease are hoarseness, stridor and aspiration.

Chapter 32

Laryngotracheal trauma

The larynx and trachea may be injured by

- penetrating wounds, e.g. gunshot or knife injuries (Fig. 32.1)
- blunt trauma, especially from road traffic accidents
- inhaled flames or hot vapours
- swallowed corrosive poisons
- endotracheal tubes and inflatable cuffs (iatrogenic injury).

Management

The diagnosis of laryngotracheal trauma is often missed amid other serious injuries. Consider it when the neck is injured. Fractures of the larynx will produce hoarseness and stridor, and urgent tracheostomy may be needed. In cases of cut

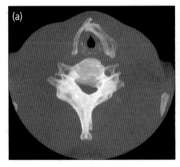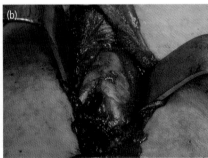

Figure 32.1 CT scan and operation showing fracture of the thyroid cartilage and the result of repair by wiring. The patient was a medical student, injured in rugby training.

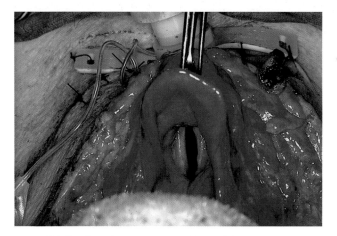

Figure 32.2 A self-inflicted cut throat, giving a good view of the anatomy.

throat, it may be possible to intubate the larynx through the wound, prior to formal tracheostomy and laryngeal repair. The immediate priority is to establish an airway by intubation or tracheostomy (Fig. 32.2). Laryngeal repair may be needed later.

Laryngeal stenosis may result and a permanent tracheostomy is sometimes necessary.

Iatrogenic laryngotracheal injuries

Long-term endotracheal intubation of patients on intensive care units can cause ischaemia of the laryngotracheal mucosa and long-term scarring. This can reduce and permanently scar the airway, especially in children where the tracheal lumen is in any case narrow. Prolonged endotracheal ventilation for broncho-pulmonary dysplasia and respiratory distress syndrome has inevitably resulted in cases of laryngeal stenosis in tiny infants, especially premature babies. More recently, the avoidance of irritant rubber tubes, awareness of the need to control cuff pressures and a tendency to use smaller calibre endotracheal tubes have led to a reduction in the incidence of airway stenosis.

Clinical practice point

- Always look for signs of laryngotracheal trauma in a patient with neck injuries.

Chapter 33

Inflammatory disorders of the larynx

Acute laryngitis: adults

Clinical features

- Aphonia (the voice is lost or reduced to a whisper).
Or
- Dysphonia (hoarseness).
- Cough – sometimes painful.
- Stridor – rare but potentially serious.

Examination by indirect laryngoscopy shows a red swollen larynx, sometimes with stringy mucus between the cords.

Aetiology

Acute laryngitis is more common in the winter months. It is usually caused by a virus, e.g. acute coryza (common cold). Predisposing factors are over-use of the voice, smoking (active or passive) and alcohol.

Treatment

- Total voice rest (very difficult in practice).
- Inhalations with steam.
- Avoid smoking (active and passive).

Antibiotics are rarely needed.

Acute laryngotracheobronchitis or 'croup' in children

Acute laryngotracheobronchitis (ALTB) or 'croup' is very common in the winter months, especially in children under 2 years old. As a result of an acute viral upper respiratory infection, the laryngeal and tracheobronchial mucosa becomes swollen and oedematous. The child is unwell, typically with a harsh 'croupy' cough and a hoarse voice. Progressive airway obstruction can follow. The prognosis in ALTB or 'croup' is much better now that steroids are routinely used in the primary care management.

Treatment

- Oral steroids: dexamethasone 0.6 mg/kg. This can also be given subcutaneously or intravenously.
- Nebulized ventolin, typically 1 mL of 1 in 1000 in 3 mL of saline, or nebulized adrenaline (epinephrine) 2 mL of 1 in 1000 in 2 mL normal saline improves breathing.
- Humidification/a steamy environment soothes the harsh cough.
- Paracetamol is good analgesic and antipyretic.
- Some children will need hospital admission and rarely endotracheal intubation.

Acute epiglottitis (children)

Acute epiglottitis is a localized infection of the upper part of the larynx usually caused by *Haemophilus influenza type B (HIB)*. It causes severe swelling of the epiglottis, which obstructs the laryngeal inlet. In children it constitutes a most urgent emergency – the child may progress from being perfectly well to being dead within the space of a few hours due to airway obstruction. Fortunately, acute epiglottitis has now become very rare in the UK because of the widespread use of HIB vaccine. Sporadic cases still occur and occasionally a similar clinical picture can be caused by other organisms, e.g. *Staphylococcus*. Worldwide, in areas where the HIB vaccine is not widely used, acute epiglottitis is still a major cause of acute airway obstruction in children.

Clinical features

- The child is unwell, with increasing dysphagia.
- Drooling.
- A 'quack-like' cough.
- Stridor develops rapidly. The child will sit up, leaning forward to ease his airway.

Management of suspected acute epiglottitis

- Do not persist in examining the child's throat. You may cause spasm.
- Admit the child to hospital at once.
- Give intravenous antibiotics (amoxycillin).
- Most cases are now managed by endotracheal intubation.
- Some children will need tracheostomy.

Adult epiglottitis in adults ('supraglottitis')

In adults the pain is severe and is worsened on swallowing. It is slower to develop and to resolve than in children. Respiratory obstruction is less likely but hospital admission is still wise.

Laryngeal diphtheria

Laryngeal diphtheria is now rare in the western world. The child is ill and usually presents with a membrane on the pharynx. Stridor suggests the spread of the membrane to the larynx and trachea. Hospital admission, antitoxin and general supportive measures can be life-saving. The child may need a tracheotomy.

Chronic laryngitis

Hoarseness is a serious sign and if it persists the larynx needs to be inspected by an ENT surgeon with a view to a biopsy.

Smoking, alcohol and habitual shouting/faulty voice production can cause chronic inflammatory changes in the laryngeal mucosa. Professional voice users, e.g. teachers, actors, singers, are especially susceptible to laryngitis and may develop dysphonia due to laryngeal muscle imbalance.

The voice is hoarse and fatigues easily. There may be discomfort and a tendency to clear the throat.

Dysplasia with disorganized mucosal cellular architecture may supervene upon chronic laryngitis. In severe cases, especially if the patient continues to smoke, this can go on to cause carcinoma.

Treatment

- The voice should be rested.
- Treat upper airway sepsis.
- Steam inhalations give good symptomatic relief. Smoking is prohibited.
- Voice therapy or the support of a singing teacher may be helpful.

Chronic granulomatous laryngitis

Tuberculosis of the larynx is now very rare and occurs only in the presence of pulmonary tuberculosis. Treatment is by antituberculous drugs.

Syphilitic laryngitis is also extremely rare.

Clinical practice points

- Oral steroid therapy has greatly improved the management of ALTB or 'croup' in children.
- Acute epiglottitis is now rare in the West but still potentially fatal. Admit suspected children urgently to hospital.
- Hoarseness may be a sign of serious laryngeal disease. If it persists the larynx needs to be inspected by an ENT surgeon with a view to a biopsy.

Chapter 34

Head and neck cancer

These tumours are far less common than lung, breast and colorectal cancers but are an important cause of morbidity and mortality especially in men.

Head and neck tumours may arise from the mucosal surfaces of the aerodigestive tract – usually squamous cell carcinoma (SCC) – or from the solid organs of the head and neck, e.g. the thyroid and parathyroid glands, the salivary glands and the lymph nodes.

SCC is the commonest and the larynx is the site most often involved. The larynx, the pharynx, the oral cavity, and the nose and sinus can be the site of origin of SCC.

Even if non-fatal, head and neck cancer can have a devastating impact on patients' lives as both the disease and the treatment can affect the ability to speak, swallow and breathe. Surgery, especially if it involves the larynx, mouth and tongue, can be mutilating and may require the replacement of important structures with 'flaps' including composite grafts from other parts of the body, e.g. the forearm and lower limb. Some patients will require permanent tracheostomy or laryngectomy. The management of head and neck cancer is a subspeciality within ENT and these patients are nowadays usually looked after in designated cancer units where there is access to support facilities such as speech and language therapy, palliative care and plastic and reconstructive techniques.

Risk factors

Risk factors for SCC of the head and neck are:
- Smoking.
- Male sex.

- Older age groups.
- Lower socio-economic groups.
- Alcohol abuse.
- Betel nut chewing – popular in some communities, especially South Asia, where it causes mouth cancers.

Presentation

This depends on the site but typical clinical features are:
- Hoarseness (laryngeal cancer).
- Dysphagia (cancer of the pharynx).
- Non-healing ulcer – mouth and tongue cancer.
- Neck mass.

Disease spread and staging

SCC spreads locally and to the regional lymph nodes in the neck (loco-regional spread). Distant metastases are rare and occur late in the disease. Cancer units now use the TNM staging system to plan treatment and to compare results between centres. T (1–4) refers to the primary tumour, e.g. a small laryngeal tumour with no local spread is T1, an advanced tumour spread beyond the larynx is T4. N (0–3) refers to lymph nodes, N0 means no lymph node disease and N3 large nodes with advanced disease. M (0 or 1) refers to the presence (1) or absence (0) of distant metastases. A T1 N0 M0 tumour is therefore the earliest to present and the easiest to treat.

Treatment principles and prognosis

SCC is highly sensitive to radiation, hence early detection and good local control of disease by **radiotherapy** is the mainstay of treatment for most SCCs. Head and neck cancer patients are usually considered disease free after 2 years as unlike many mucosal cancers distant metastases are uncommon and good loco-regional control equates to cure. **Surgery** may be needed for more advanced disease, for recurrence after radiotherapy or where the neck nodes are involved. In advanced disease the support of a skilled **palliative care** team may be invaluable. **Chemotherapy** has a very limited role.

SCC of the larynx

This is the commonest site for SCC in the head and neck. Cancer may develop on the vocal cords (glottic, Fig. 34.1) above the cords (supraglottic) or below (subglottic). Glottic is the commonest and typically presents early with hoarseness. This

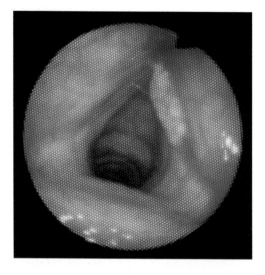

Figure 34.1 Early glottic carcinoma.

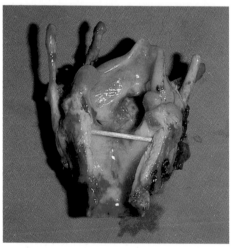

Figure **34.2** Laryngectomy specimen opened from posteriorly, showing a left-sided carcinoma.

is a curable condition with a 90% 2 year survival after radiotherapy. Some units undertake limited surgery ('cordectomy') for this disease. Supraglottic tumours present later. Subglottic tumours may present with severe airway obstruction.

Some patients with SCC of the larynx will require surgery, e.g. if there is extensive neck disease, T3 or T4 disease or recurrence after radiotherapy. A total laryngectomy (Figs 34.2 and 34.3) will mean the patient will breathe permanently through a laryngeal 'stoma'. Many patients can learn to speak by using a valve which directs expired air from the trachea into the oesophagus and pharynx (Fig. 34.4). Some

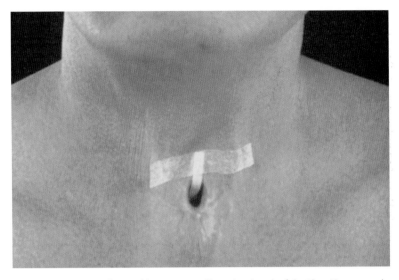

Figure 34.3 A patient after total laryngectomy. Note also the tab of the Blom Singer speech valve.

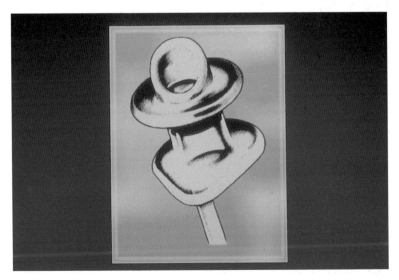

Figure 34.4 A 'Blom Singer' valve to facilitate speech after a total laryngectomy. The valve permits air to flow from the trachea to the oesophagus.

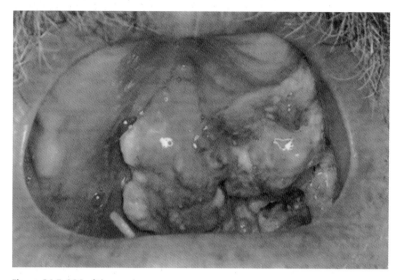

Figure 34.5 SCC of the oropharynx.

patients develop the ability to vibrate the oesophagus without a valve (oesophageal speech).

SCC of the pharynx and oral cavity

SCC of the pharynx is less common than laryngeal cancer with a worse prognosis. Any part of the pharynx may be affected. **Nasopharyngeal** cancer primarily occurs in Chinese men and is considered in Chapter 25. **Oropharyngeal** cancer (Fig. 34.5) typically involves the tonsils (Chapter 29). The '**hypopharynx**' or lowerpart of the pharynx, i.e. as it enters the oesophagus, is adjacent to the larynx and cancer here has a particularly poor prognosis. Presentation may be with dysphagia, hoarseness or both. Neck metastases are a particularly bad sign. **Oral cavity** tumours often present as non-healing ulcers and may be treated by excision – sometimes needing extensive flap repair – or radiotherapy depending on their extent.

Clinical practice points

- The main presentations for head and neck cancer are hoarseness, dysphagia, a neck mass and a non-healing ulcer in the mouth or pharynx. Patients with any of these for 2 weeks or more should be considered for urgent ENT referral.
- Early detection of SCC is vital and greatly improves survival.
- Radiotherapy is the mainstay of treatment for SCC of the head and neck.

Chapter 35

Voice disorders

The larygeal musculature is an intricate system for varying the length, tension and degree of apposition of the vocal cords. Conditions which affect the laryngeal mucosa or the laryngeal nerves and muscles cause hoarseness (dysphonia) with, in severe cases, aphonia (no voice). Voice is one of the important instruments we use to express feelings and emotions, and it is wise to be sensitive to the possibility of anxiety, depression and psychological distress in patients with voice disorders. Professional voice users such as actors, singers and teachers are especially susceptible. The management of voice disorders (phoniatrics and phonosurgery) is now a subspeciality within ENT and many units will have a voice clinic run by an ENT surgeon and a speech and language therapist. Hoarseness is a serious symptom. If it persists for more than two weeks refer the patient to an ENT clinic.

'Muscle tension' dysphonia

Many voice disorders are due to incoordination of the intrinsic laryngeal musculature. The signs are subtle and only apparent on close inspection of the larynx at endoscopy using a stroboscope and with the patient using his voice. These disorders were often regarded as 'functional' dysphonias in the past and ascribed to psychological causes. Some patients do present with complete aphonia due to psychological morbidity. The help of a speech and language therapist is invaluable in treating these patients and many will need several sessions of voice therapy.

Vocal cord nodules

Vocal cord nodules occur both in adults ('singer's nodes') and children ('screamer's nodules') and result from excessive vocal use. The appearance is of a small,

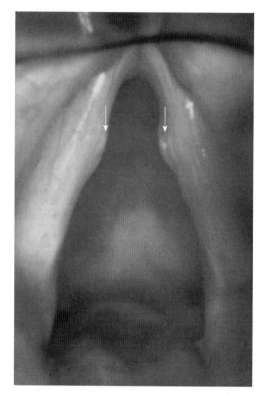

Figure 35.1 Vocal cord nodules.

smooth nodule on the free edge of each cord, composed of fibrous tissue covered with epithelium (Fig. 35.1). Most cases respond to voice rest and speech therapy. Nodules very rarely need to be removed surgically.

Vocal cord paralysis

Usually unilateral, this presents as a hoarse breathy voice as the cords are unable to appose (Figs 35.2 and 35.3). In severe cases the patient may aspirate food and saliva as one of the functions of the cords is to close the laryngeal inlet during swallowing. The muscles responsible for moving the vocal cords are in the main supplied by the recurrent laryngeal nerves. These are branches of the vagus nerve. On the left the nerve has a longer course and winds around the aortic arch in the chest before entering the neck. Hence left recurrent laryngeal nerve palsy is more common and more likely to be caused by chest pathology.

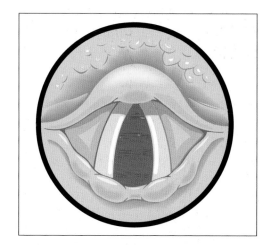

Figure 35.2 The cords in full abduction during inspiration.

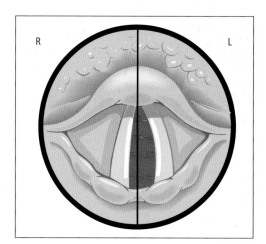

Figure 35.3 Left recurrent nerve palsy on phonation (mirror view). Note the persisting glottic aperture owing to the inability of the left cord to move to the midline.

A chest X-ray is mandatory. The recurrent laryngeal nerve can be injured anywhere from the brain stem to the chest.

Some chest causes of left recurrent nerve palsy are:

- Carcinoma of the bronchus.
- Carcinoma of the oesophagus.
- Malignant mediastinal nodes.
- Aortic aneurysm.
- Cardiac and oesophageal surgery.

The right or left recurrent nerve in the neck can easily be traumatized by thyroid surgery or involved in thyroid or other neck cancers.

Some cases of recurrent nerve palsy are idiopathic or may follow viral infections, such as influenza.

Bilateral recurrent laryngeal nerve palsy

This occurs most commonly following surgery or malignancy of the thyroid gland, but may be the result of brain stem pathology, e.g. pseudobulbar palsy. Because the cords lie near the midline, the airway is impaired. Tracheostomy may be needed.

Treatment of vocal cord paralysis

- Try to identify the cause.
- Many cases can be treated conservatively, particularly if recovery is expected.
- In 'thyroplasty' operations a window is cut in the thyroid cartilage and a block of silastic inserted to displace the cord towards the midline. It has the advantage of being reversible if the cord palsy should recover.

Clinical practice point

- Hoarseness is a serious symptom. If it persists for more than 2 weeks, refer the patient to an ENT clinic.

Chapter 36

Airway obstruction in infants and children

Upper airway obstruction (see Box 36.1) in children is dangerous and may progress rapidly. Make a firm diagnosis and take the appropriate action without delay.

Management of airway obstruction

The management of airway insufficiency always depends on the severity. Severe obstruction needs immediate airway support by oxygen, endotracheal intubation or very rarely tracheostomy.

Box 36.1 Signs of airway obstruction

- **Stertor** produced by obstruction in the throat, i.e. above the larynx, is a low-pitched choking type of noise.
- **Stridor** is a high-pitched sound produced by narrowing within the more rigid confines of the larynx or trachea. In laryngeal obstruction the stridor is inspiratory; in tracheal lesions it is usually both inspiratory and expiratory.
- Use of **accessory muscles of respiration**.
- Intercostal and sternal **recession** (Fig. 36.1). The sternum may be sucked in almost to the vertebrae in the child's attempts to breathe.
- **Pallor**, sweating and restlessness.
- **Tachycardia**.
- **Cyanosis**. Examine the child in adequate lighting, preferably daylight. The lips particularly will show the dusky colouration, which may be very subtle.
- **Exhaustion** – a late stage in asphyxia, which should be avoided. The child makes less effort to breathe, stridor and recession becomes less pronounced and apnoea is not far off.

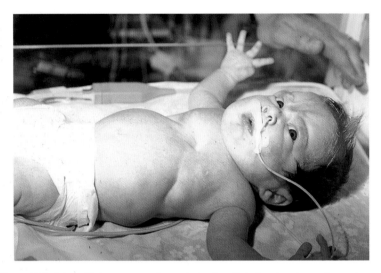

Figure 36.1 Baby with severe upper airway obstruction. Note the sternal recession and paradoxical abdominal movement.

If time and the child's condition allow, every child with stridor should have chest X-ray and a lateral soft-tissue film of the neck, which will show the larynx and upper trachea clearly. If a vascular ring or tracheo-oesophageal fistula is suspected, arrange a barium swallow.

Neonates may be intubated without the need for general anaesthesia but great care must be taken not to damage the larynx and cause further obstruction from haematoma or oedema. Older children, unless so anoxic as to be unconscious, will require general anaesthesia for intubation, and at the same time the larynx, trachea and bronchi should be inspected. The diagnosis is then usually apparent and further management can be directed appropriately.

Laryngoscopy and bronchoscopy

Inspection of the airways in cases of respiratory obstruction calls for the highest degree of cooperation between surgeon and anaesthetist.

The larynx is inspected under deep anaesthesia using a rigid paediatric laryngoscope and Hopkins rod telescope (Fig. 36.2). An anaesthetic-type laryngoscope usually gives an inadequate view owing to its poorer lighting.

Bronchoscopy in babies and children has been facilitated greatly by the introduction of ventilating bronchoscopes, which allow coupling to a T-piece anaesthetic circuit and at the same time provide superb vision through a rod-lens telescope system (Fig. 36.3). A side channel allows for instrumentation and

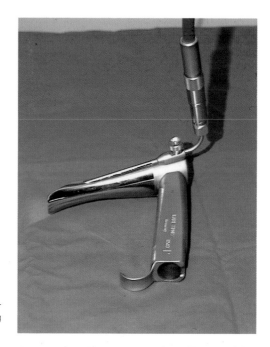

Figure 36.2 A small laryngoscope used for examining young children.

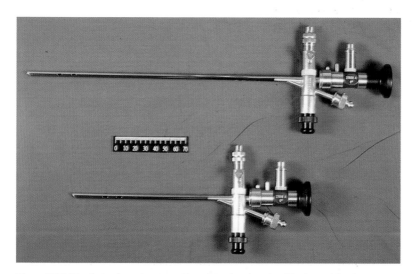

Figure 36.3 Ventilating bronchoscopes. Note the telescope, the side channel for instrumentation and the inlet for anaesthetic gases and oxygen.

suction. Using this type of bronchoscope, the airways of even small premature babies may be examined with a much greater degree of precision and safety than is possible with the older type open bronchoscope tube.

Causes of upper airway obstruction in infancy

Supralaryngeal causes

Choanal atresia

Failure of posterior canalization of the nasal airways results in severe neonatal airway obstruction, which is relieved by crying. Surgical correction will be required.

Micrognathia

Underdevelopment of the mandible as in Pierre Robin sequence (which includes cleft palate) or Treacher–Collins syndrome (see Chapter 5) results in posterior displacement of the tongue (glossoptosis) and oropharyngeal obstruction. The neonate may asphyxiate unless corrective measures – e.g. insertion of an oral airway or a nasopharyngeal tube – are taken.

Adeno-tonsillar hypertrophy

Large tonsils and adenoids may occlude the naso-oropharyngeal airway to a serious degree, especially during sleep. This may result in obstructive apnoea during sleep, with loud snoring punctuated by periods of silence followed by a large gasp. If not recognized and treated, right heart failure may ensue.

Laryngeal causes

Congenital

Laryngomalacia (floppy larynx, Fig. 36.4)
The stridor starts at or shortly after birth and is due to inward collapse of the soft laryngeal tissues on inspiration. It usually resolves by the age of 2 or 3 years, but meanwhile the baby may have real respiratory difficulties. Diagnosis is confirmed by laryngoscopy without intubation when the supraglottic collapse is seen on inspiration. It can be relieved by division or excision of the membrane between the epiglottis and the arytenoids (aryepiglottic folds).

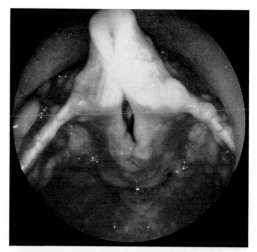

Figure 36.4 Laryngomalacia. Note the insuction of the supraglottic structures, causing airway narrowing.

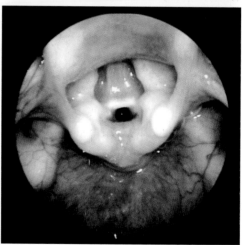

Figure 36.5 Anterior laryngeal web.

Congenital subglottic stenosis

This occurs at the level of the cricoid cartilage. There will be stridor from birth and the stenosis may be visible on a lateral X-ray of the neck. Diagnosis is confirmed by laryngoscopy.

Laryngeal webs

Laryngeal webs are usually anteriorly situated (Fig. 36.5) and if large can cause severe stridor and obstruction. The most extreme degree of webbing, atresia, is fatal without an immediate tracheostomy.

155

Laryngeal cysts

Laryngeal cysts may be congenital or may be the result of endotracheal intubation. They may cause variable airway obstruction, often dependent on position.

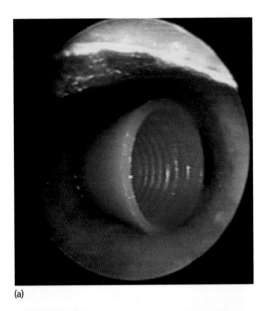

(a)

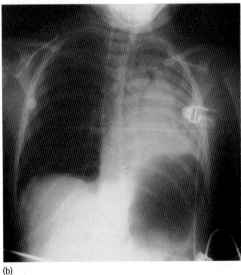

(b)

Figure 36.6 (a) Part of a ball-point pen lodged in the left main bronchus as seen at bronchoscopy. (b) The chest film shows loss of lung volume and mediastinal shift.

Vascular ring

A vascular ring – developmental anomaly of the aorta – surrounds the oesophagus and trachea, causing constriction. Diagnosis is made by barium swallow and MR scanning. Treatment is by surgery to divide the vascular ring.

Acquired

Foreign body (Figs 36.6 and 36.7)

The sudden onset of stridor in a previously healthy child must always be regarded as due to a foreign body until proved otherwise. A history of choking and coughing, especially while eating, should alert the attending doctor to the likelihood of aspiration; peanuts are particularly dangerous in this respect and should *never* be given to youngsters. A foreign body in the bronchus may permit some air entry but obstruct it mainly in expiration. This can cause a 'ball valve' effect with hyperinflation of one lung on chest X-ray – the so-called 'obstructive emphysema' (Fig 36.7). However examination and chest X-rays may be entirely normal and the only way to exclude a foreign body in the bronchus is by bronchoscopy.

A larger foreign body may lodge in the larynx and cause severe respiratory distress. It may be possible to remove it by the Heimlich manoeuvre (compression of the upper abdomen to raise intrathoracic pressure) but if this fails, endoscopy or tracheostomy will be necessary.

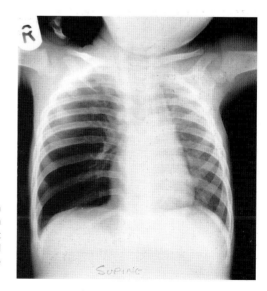

Figure 36.7 Foreign body in the right main bronchus in a baby of 6 months. Note that the right lung is hyperinflated and therefore darker on the X-ray.

Acute laryngitis, acute epiglottitis and laryngotracheobronchitis

Described in Chapter 33.

Subglottic stenosis (Fig. 36.8)

Subglottic stenosis is now seen most commonly in low-birth-weight babies who have required prolonged ventilation by endotracheal tube, but may occur at any age from intubation or trauma. Treatment is highly specialized and entails some form of laryngotracheoplasty to reconstruct the airway. Subglottic stenosis cannot always be avoided.

Recurrent respiratory papillomatosis (Fig. 36.9)

This is a serious condition caused by the human papilloma virus (HPV) types 6 and 11. The virus is thought to be transmitted through the mother's birth

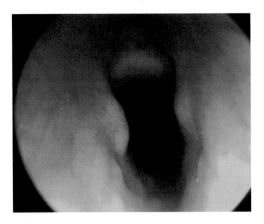

Figure 36.8 Endoscopic view showing moderate subglottic stenosis and small ductal cysts following ventilation as a neonate.

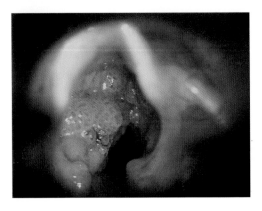

Figure 36.9 A large mass of papillomata on the left vocal cord.

canal. Suspect papillomatosis in a child with progressive hoarseness or aphonia and airway obstruction. There may be little stridor since the mass of papillomas is too soft to vibrate the air column. Diagnosis is by direct laryngoscopy. Removal of the papillomas is best accomplished using a microdebrider at laryngotracheoscopy. The papillomas have a strong tendency to recur.

Clinical practice points

- Any child with stridor is potentially at risk of dying from asphyxia. Every case should be investigated to determine the cause. It is dangerous to believe that all children 'grow out' of a tendency to stridor.
- Beware the exhausted child whose stridor has quietened. He may be near asphyxiation.
- Never allow young children near peanuts or other small objects they may inhale and advise parents and carers accordingly. An inhaled foreign body can be fatal.

Chapter 37

The pharynx

Ingested foreign bodies

Children, adults with learning disabilities and patients with psychiatric morbidity may ingest coins, toys or more bizarre objects (Fig. 37.1). If inhaled they may be expelled by coughing. More seriously they may cause airway obstruction or impact in a bronchus (see Chapter 36). Some will impact in the pharynx or oesophagus. Elderly patients may swallow their dentures. Sometimes poorly chewed food – especially a bolus of meat – can obstruct the oesophagus. Fish, poultry and other bones are often inadvertently swallowed. They may scratch or tear the pharyngeal mucosa before passing down into the stomach. They can also

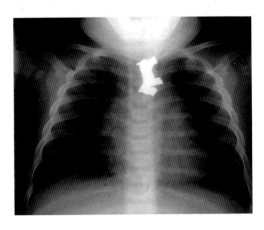

Figure 37.1 Man eats dog.

lodge in the pharynx or oesophagus, where they may lead to perforation, mediastinitis or abscess, or even fatal perforation of the aorta. The potential gravity of an impacted foreign body cannot be over-emphasized.

Sharp foreign body

If a patient presents with a history of having swallowed a sharp foreign body – e.g. a bone – he will complain of soreness in the throat. It may be very difficult to decide whether a foreign body has simply caused an abrasion and has passed on, or is impacted. Adopt the following routine:
• Take a careful history, noting the nature of the suspected foreign body (is it radio-opaque?) and the time of ingestion.
• Examine the pharynx and larynx. Pay particular attention to the tonsils and tongue base. (Fish bones often stick here.) A foreign body lodged in the cervical oesophagus will cause pain on gently pressing the larynx against the spine.
• X-ray the chest and neck (lateral view) – remember that plastic and some fish bones will not show.
• If there is any doubt, seek expert advice.
    Indications for pharyngo-oesophagoscopy are:
• Dysphagia.
• Suspected foreign body on X-ray.
• Persistent symptoms.

Impacted food bolus

Dysphagia and drooling suggest complete oesophageal obstruction. A carbonated drink may help, as may a gentle sedative such as intravenous diazepam. If the bolus has impacted, admission to hospital and endoscopic removal will be needed.

Post-cricoid web

The Paterson–Brown Kelly syndrome (later described by Plummer and Vinson) is associated with iron-deficiency anaemia and the development of a pharyngeal ('post-cricoid') web causing dysphagia. The features of iron deficiency (glossitis, angular stomatitis and microcytic anaemia) will be present. The web can be demonstrated by barium swallow.

The iron deficiency is corrected by iron supplements and the web is dilated periodically. A small number of patients with this condition will go on to develop pharyngeal carcinoma.

Pharyngeal pouch ('hypopharyngeal diverticulum')

The pharyngeal mucosa herniates between the oblique and transverse fibres of the inferior constrictor muscle to produce a persistent pouch (Fig. 37.2). The condition occurs mostly in the elderly and is thought to be due to failure of the cricopharyngeus part of the inferior constrictor to relax during swallowing, thus building up pressure above it.

Clinical features

- Discomfort in the throat.
- Dysphagia as the pouch enlarges.
- Regurgitation of undigested food.
- Aspiration pneumonia.
- If the pouch is large, gurgling noises in the throat on swallowing.
- A pouch almost never causes a palpable neck swelling.

Investigation

The pouch is seen on barium swallow (Fig. 37.2).

Treatment

An established pouch causing symptoms will require surgical treatment. Under general anaesthesia, a dilating rigid pharyngoscope is used to demonstrate the party wall between the oesophagus anteriorly and the pouch posteriorly. A staple gun is then used to divide the wall and at the same time staple the cut edges (Fig. 37.3). The patient is usually able to eat the following day and the hospital stay is very short.

It is now rarely necessary to excise a pouch by external approach through the neck.

Globus pharyngeus

The sensation of a 'lump in the throat' is familiar to everyone and occurs during periods of heightened emotion. It is probably due to tightening of the cricopharyngeus muscle which separates the pharynx from the oesophagus. Many patients complain bitterly of a sensation of a 'lump' or discomfort in the throat, sometimes intermittent and sometimes constant. **Globus pharyngeus** is the term applied to this sensation. The discomfort is often relieved by eating. There is no interference with swallowing of food or liquids.

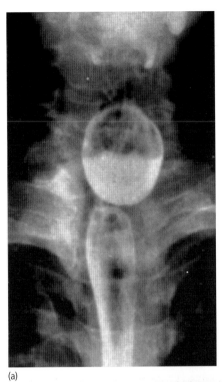

(a)

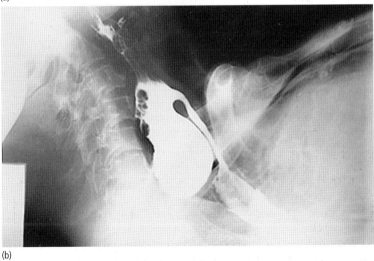

(b)

Figure 37.2 A barium swallow X-ray showing a pharyngeal pouch (a) and lateral view (b).

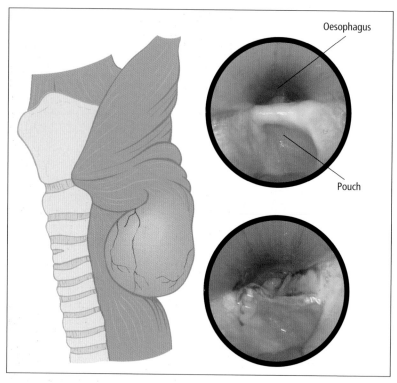

Oesophagus

Pouch

Figure 37.3 External and endoscopic views of the pharyngeal pouch. The photographs show appearances before and after endoscopic diverticulotomy with a stapling device.

Symptoms tend to be aggravated by the patient's constant action of swallowing, and frequently introspection and anxiety add to the problem. A proportion of patients with globus pharyngeus will have reflux oesophagitis but whether this association is causal or not is debated. Many patients develop anxiety that they have developed throat cancer and if symptoms persist thorough endoscopy is essential.

Most patients improve with reassurance reinforced by adequate examination and investigation but for many this is a troublesome and recalcitrant condition. Older text-books describe this condition as 'globus hystericus' reflecting its alleged psychological aetiology and its increased prevalence in women but most patients have no psychological morbidity. Men are frequently affected.

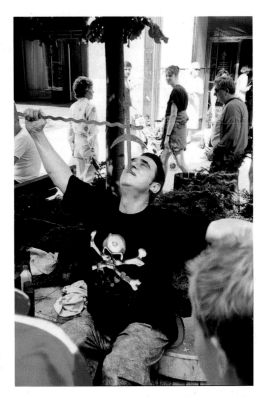

Figure 37.4 A sword swallower in Prague. The first ever oesophagoscopy was performed in the 19th century on a sword swallower by Küssmaul to demonstrate its feasibility.

Clinical practice points

- An ingested foreign body is potentially serious. Seek help if in any doubt.
- Globus pharyngeus is now the commonest reason for referral to an adult ENT clinic. Most patients respond to reassurance.

Chapter 38

Tracheostomy

Tracheostomy, the making of an opening into the trachea, has been practised since the first century BC. It can be life-saving and all doctors should know something of it.

Indications for tracheostomy

- To bypass upper airway obstruction.
- To protect the tracheobronchial tree.
- To facilitate artificial ventilation.

Protection of the tracheobronchial tube

Any condition causing pharyngeal or laryngeal incompetence may allow aspiration of food, saliva, blood or gastric contents. If the condition is of short duration, e.g. general anaesthesia, endotracheal intubation is best, but for chronic conditions tracheostomy may be needed. This allows easy access to the trachea and bronchi for regular suction and permits the use of a cuffed tube, which further protects against aspiration. Examples of such conditions are:

Neurological disorders, e.g. polyneuritis (e.g. Guillain–Barré syndrome), brain stem stroke.

Coma if it is likely to be prolonged, e.g. due to:

- head injury,
- poisoning,
- stroke.

Upper airway obstruction

Congenital
- Subglottic or upper tracheal stenosis.
- Laryngeal web.
- Laryngeal cysts/haemangioma.
- Tracheo-oesophageal anomalies.

Trauma
- Prolonged endotracheal intubation.
- Gunshot wounds and cut throat, laryngeal fracture.
- Inhalation/corrosive injury.
- Radiotherapy (may cause oedema).

Infections
- Acute epiglottitis (see Chapter 33).
- Laryngotracheobronchitis.
- Diphtheria.
- Ludwig's angina.

Malignant tumours
- Advanced malignant disease of the tongue, larynx, pharynx or upper trachea.
- As part of a surgical procedure for the treatment of laryngeal cancer.
- Thyroid carcinoma.

Bilateral laryngeal paralysis
- Following thyroidectomy.
- Bulbar palsy.
- Following oesophageal or heart surgery.

Foreign body in the airway
Remember the Heimlich manoeuvre – grasp the patient from behind with a fist in the epigastrium and apply sudden pressure upwards towards the diaphragm. It may need to be repeated several times before the foreign body is expelled.

To facilitate artificial ventilation

If ventilation is to be for a long period, tracheostomy is preferable to an endotracheal tube.

Tracheostomy in cases of respiratory failure allows:
- Reduction of dead space by about 70 mL (in the adult).
- Bypass of laryngeal resistance.
- Access to the trachea for the removal of bronchial secretions.
- Administration of humidified oxygen.
- Positive-pressure ventilation when necessary.

Tracheostomy should, whenever possible, be carried out as an elective procedure and not as a desperate last resort. There are degrees of urgency.

Life-threatening airway obstruction

If endotracheal intubation fails or is impossible, tracheostomy must be done at once. There is no time for sterility – with the left hand, hold the trachea on either side to immobilize it, make a vertical incision through the tissues of the neck into the trachea and twist the blade through 90° to open up the trachea. There will be copious dark bleeding but the patient will gasp air through the opening. Using the index finger of the left hand as a guide in the wound, try to insert some sort of tube into the trachea. The blood should then be sucked out by whatever means are available. Once an airway is established, the tracheostomy can be tidied up under more controlled conditions. If you are unable to do a tracheostomy as described you can buy a little time until more experienced help is available by inserting a wide-bore needle into the cricothyroid membrane (Fig. 38.1).

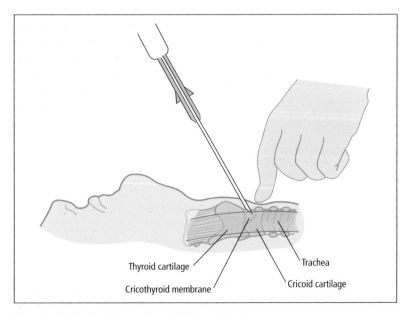

Thyroid cartilage

Cricothyroid membrane

Trachea

Cricoid cartilage

Figure 38.1 Cricothyroidotomy (from APLS manual).

Airway obstruction of more gradual onset

Do not allow the situation to deteriorate to that described above. Stridor, recession and tachycardia denote the need for intervention, and cyanosis and bradycardia indicate that you are running out of time. The case should be discussed with an experienced anaesthetist, and the patient taken to the operating theatre. The ideal is to carry out tracheostomy under general anaesthesia with endotracheal intubation. Once a tube has been inserted, the airway is safe and the tracheostomy can be performed calmly and carefully with full sterile precautions. If the anaesthetist is unable to intubate the patient, it will be necessary to perform the operation under local anaesthetic using infiltration with lignocaine. The anaesthetist meanwhile will administer oxygen through a face mask.

Elective tracheostomy

Like any other operation, tracheostomy can be learned only by instruction and practice. Only a brief description is given.

Tracheostomy is best done under general anaesthesia with endotracheal intubation. The neck should be extended and the head must be straight, not turned to one side. A transverse incision is preferable to a vertical incision, and should be centred midway between the cricoid cartilage and sternal notch (Fig. 38.2). The strap muscles are identified and retracted laterally (Fig. 38.3) and the thyroid isthmus is divided. Once the trachea has been reached (it is always deeper than you expect), the cricoid must be identified by palpation and the tracheal rings counted. An opening is made into the trachea, centred on the third and fourth rings (Fig. 38.4). A single slit in the tracheal wall is best, after first inserting stay sutures on either side to allow traction on the opening in order to insert the tube.

After insertion of the tracheostomy tube, the trachea is aspirated thoroughly. The skin incision is left unsutured.

After-care of the tracheostomy

Nursing care

Nursing care must be of the highest standard to keep the tube patent and prevent dislodgement.

Position

Adult patients in the post-operative period should usually be sitting well propped up; take care in infants that the chin does not occlude the tracheostomy; extend the baby's neck slightly over a rolled-up towel.

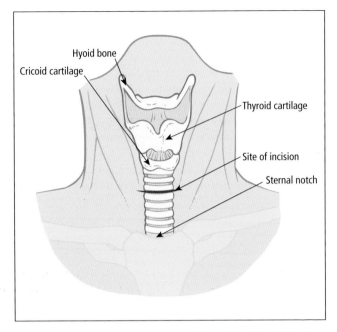

Figure 38.2 Tracheostomy showing the landmarks of the neck and the incision for operation.

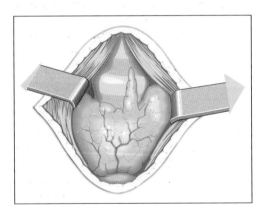

Figure 38.3 The strap muscles are retracted, exposing the trachea and the thyroid isthmus.

Suction

Suction is applied at regular intervals dictated by the amount of secretions present. A clean catheter must be passed down into the tube in conscious patients. Unconscious or ventilated patients will require deeper suction and physiotherapy.

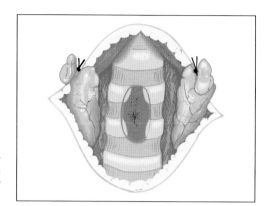

Figure 38.4 The thyroid isthmus has been divided and an opening made in the anterior tracheal wall.

Humidification

Humidification of the inspired air is essential to prevent drying and the formation of crusts. If necessary, sterile saline (1 mL) can be introduced into the trachea, followed by suction.

Tube changing

Tube changing should be avoided if possible for 2 or 3 days, after which the track should be well established and the tube can be changed easily. Cuffed tubes need particular attention, with regular deflation of the cuff to prevent pressure necrosis. The amount of air in the cuff should be the minimum required to prevent an air leak.

Decannulation

Decannulation should only be carried out when it is obvious that the tracheostomy is no longer required. The patient should be able to manage with the tube occluded for at least 24 h before it is removed (Fig. 38.5).

Decannulation in children often presents particular difficulties. After decannulation, the patient should remain in hospital under observation for several days.

Complications

- **Bleeding**.
- **Pneumothorax**. Due to perforation of the pleura. This usually heals but may make post-operative care very difficult. Mediastinal emphysema can also occur.

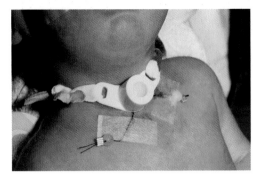

Figure 38.5 A newly performed tracheostomy in a small child. Note the stay sutures on either side to aid replacement of the tube should it become dislodged.

- **Obstruction** of the tube or trachea by crusts of inspissated secretion may be fatal. Act boldly, remove the whole tube and replace it if blocked. If the tube is patent, explore the trachea with angled forceps to remove the obstruction. An explosive cough may expel the crust and the tube can then be replaced.

- **Complete dislodgement** of the tube if it is not adequately fixed. Hold the wound edges apart with a tracheal dilator and put in a clean tube. Good light is essential.

- **Partial dislodgement** of the tube is more difficult to recognize and may be fatal. The tube comes to lie in front of the trachea, the airway will be impaired and, if left, erosion of the innominate artery may result in catastrophic haemorrhage. Make sure that at all times the patient breathes freely through the tube.

- **Surgical emphysema** may occur if the patient is on positive-pressure ventilation. It is usually self-limiting.

- **Perichondritis and subglottic stenosis** especially if the cricoid cartilage is injured. Go below the first ring.

Clinical practice points

- In respiratory obstruction or respiratory failure if there is no steady improvement, support the airway by endotracheal intubation or tracheostomy.
- Learn the technique of emergency tracheostomy/cricothyroidotomy.
- Remember that children may deteriorate very quickly.

Chapter 39

Diseases of the salivary glands

Applied basic science

The salivary glands consist of:
- The parotid glands.
- The submandibular glands.
- Minor salivary glands throughout the mouth and upper air passages. (The sublingual collection is included in this group.)

Parotid gland

The parotid gland lies on the side of the face in close relationship to the ear, the angle of the mandible and styloid muscles. The facial nerve enters the posterior pole of the parotid gland and divides within its substance into its various branches, which exit at the anterior margin of the gland. It is the presence of the facial nerve within the parotid that makes surgery of this gland so difficult. Its duct opens opposite the second upper molar tooth, where it forms a small visible papilla. Its secretomotor nerve supply comes from the glossopharyngeal nerve via the tympanic plexus in the middle ear.

The saliva produced is entirely serous. The surface outline of the gland is shown in Fig. 39.1.

The submandibular salivary gland

The submandibular gland lies in the floor of the mouth below and medial to the mandible. It is mostly below the mylohyoid muscle which forms the floor of

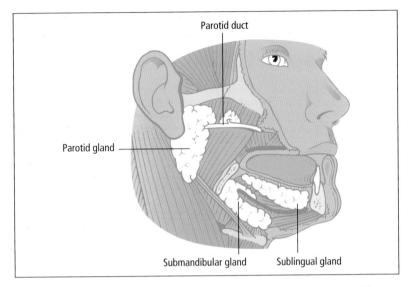

Parotid duct

Parotid gland

Submandibular gland   Sublingual gland

Figure 39.1 The surface outline of the parotid and submandibular glands. The parotid gland is larger than is usually appreciated.

the mouth. The deep part of the gland curves around the back of the mylohyoid and the duct runs forward to open at the sublingual papilla, one on either side of the midline. The deep part of the gland lies on the lingual nerve, from which it receives its secretomotor supply derived from the facial nerve via the chorda tympani in the middle ear. The saliva from the submandibular gland is both serous and mucous.

The minor salivary glands

The minor salivary glands can be seen and felt in the lips, cheeks, palate and upper air passages. They produce mainly mucous saliva and are responsible for a large proportion of the total saliva secreted. They are subject to many of the diseases that affect the major salivary glands.

History-taking

- Enquire about pain and swelling of the glands in relation to eating. If the duct is obstructed, the whole gland will become tense and painful and enlarge visibly during saliva production, and will reduce slowly over about an hour.
- If there is a lump, ask about variation in size and whether it is related to food. Tumours do not enlarge during salivation, but do tend to get bigger with the passage of time.

174

- Ask about dryness of the mouth, remembering that obstruction of even two major glands produces little apparent change. Persistent dryness suggests diffuse salivary gland disease.
- Ask about recent contact with mumps.

Examination of the salivary glands

- Inspect the salivary glands externally, noting any swellings or asymmetry. Test the function of the facial nerve in all its divisions.
- Inspect the parotid and submandibular ducts to assess saliva flow, redness and the presence of pus or an obvious stone. Inspect the mouth to see if it is excessively dry.
- Palpate the glands. In the case of the submandibular gland put one gloved finger into the mouth as you feel the gland externally (bimanual palpation). Feel for calculi especially at the duct orifices.
- If the patient is given an acid-drop to suck any enlargement on salivation can be assessed.
- Check the ears.
- Examine the rest of the neck for lymph nodes.

Investigation

- Plain X-ray, including occlusal views, will show a radio-opaque calculus.
- Ultrasonic scanning is quick, non-invasive and safe. Good for masses and cysts.
- CT/MRI. If there is a large parotid tumour an MR scan will outline it well.
- Sialography. Contrast medium injected into the gland after cannulation of the duct. Invasive, less often used nowadays.

Inflammation of the salivary glands (sialadenitis)

Mumps

Mumps is the commonest acute inflammatory condition of salivary glands. Infection is with the mumps virus. It affects mainly the parotid glands, which become uniformly swollen and painful, but the submandibular glands may also be involved. Its incidence had fallen to very low levels as a result of immunization, but is now rising alarmingly as some parents decline to have their children immunized. Mumps parotitis is self-limiting and managed with analgesics but complications can include deafness, orchitis with the risk of infertility in boys, and encephalitis.

Acute suppurative parotitis

This is uncommon and usually occurs in debilitated patients. Treatment is with antibiotics, rehydration and oral hygiene. An abscess may need surgical incision.

Acute sialadenitis

Acute sialadenitis may affect the submandibular gland (commonly) or the parotid gland (rarely) because of the presence of a duct calculus. The patient is usually unwell with a fever. The affected gland is painful and swollen and is made worse by eating. Removal of the stone provides dramatic relief in most cases.

Recurrent acute inflammation

Recurrent acute inflammation of the major salivary glands presents a problem of management if there is no stone. In childhood, recurrent episodes of acute inflammation will usually subside by puberty. Treat conservatively.

Chronic inflammation

Chronic inflammation of the parotid or submandibular gland is usually due to sialectasis (duct dilatation leading to stasis and infection). The gland is thickened with episodic pain and infection, and can be felt easily on bimanual examination.

The submandibular gland so affected can be excised; chronic sialectasis of the parotid poses a difficult problem. Excision has a high risk of facial nerve damage and long-term antibiotics should be tried before resorting to parotidectomy.

Sjögren's syndrome

Sjögren's syndrome is an auto-immune systemic disorder affecting the salivary and lacrimal glands. There is enlargement of the glands and loss of secretion, leading to dryness of the eyes and mouth. Symptomatic relief can be obtained by the use of artificial saliva or glycerine and warm-water mouthwash.

Salivary retention cysts

Salivary cysts occur most commonly in the floor of the mouth, where they may become very large and expand the loose tissues (Fig. 39.2). The name 'ranula' is often applied. Less commonly, such retention cysts occur on the mucosal aspect of the lips.

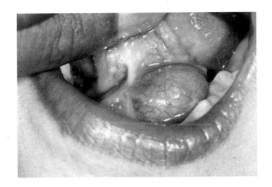

Figure 39.2 Sublingual retention cyst.

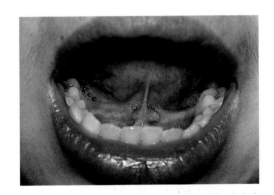

Figure 39.3 Calculus in left submandibular duct orifice.

Salivary calculi

Most salivary calculi occur in the submandibular gland because of the mucoid nature of its saliva, which can become inspissated (Fig. 39.3). However, calculi do also occur in the parotid gland.

Clinical features

The flow of saliva from the affected gland becomes obstructed, causing the gland to swell during salivation. Such swelling is painful and its size may be alarming. The swelling will usually resolve over about an hour.

The calculus can be seen if it presents at the duct opening, or felt within the duct or gland.

Investigation

Most calculi are radio-opaque and will show on plain X-ray.

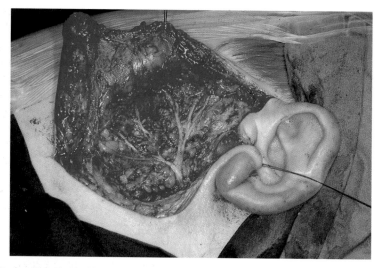

Figure 39.4 The facial nerve after superficial parotidectomy for a benign tumour in a boy aged 12 years.

Treatment

Intraductal calculi can be removed from the duct under local anaesthetic. If the stone is within the substance of the salivary gland, excision of the gland may be best. The submandibular gland is straightforward to excise, but parotidectomy requires a high degree of skill (Fig. 39.4).

Salivary gland tumours

Salivary glands contain lymph nodes within their structure and may be the site of metastases from a non-salivary primary site or from blood dyscrasias such as leukaemia (Fig. 39.5). Primary tumours of the salivary glands are uncommon.

Benign tumours

- Pleomorphic salivary adenoma (mixed salivary tumour, PSA) (Fig. 39.6). By far the commonest. Most frequently in the parotid gland. Tend to recur if not removed with surrounding cuff of tissue. PSA accounts for about 90% of parotid tumours in adults.
- Warthin's tumour (cystic lymphoepithelial lesion).
- Haemangioma.

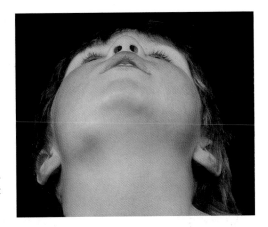

Figure 39.5 Enlarged right sub-mandibular gland from chronic infection.

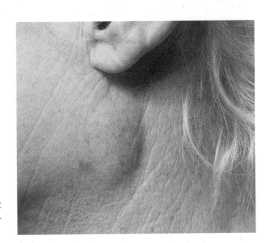

Figure 39.6 A pleomorphic adenoma in the tail of the parotid gland.

Malignant tumours

- Adenoid cystic carcinoma. The commonest malignant tumour of salivary glands. With early perineural invasion, the long-term prognosis is poor but survival for many years is usual.
- Muco-epidermoid tumours.
- Acinic cell tumours.
- Malignant pleomorphic adenomata.
- Squamous carcinoma.

Lymphoma

May be benign or malignant. The lymphoma arises from lymphoid tissue within any of the salivary glands.

Drooling

While not due to disease of the salivary glands, children or adults with, for example, cerebral palsy or stroke may be unable to control the saliva produced, particularly from the sublingual and submandibular ducts. This causes much distress and discomfort to patient and relatives. Salivary flow can be reduced by the use of hyoscine patches. The patient can also be helped by surgical relocation of the submandibular ducts to divert salivary flow. The ducts are repositioned near the tonsil and the sublingual glands are excised.

Clinical practice points

- If a submandibular gland swelling gets bigger on eating, think of a stone in the submandibular duct.
- Parotid gland surgery is made particularly challenging because the facial nerve runs through the gland. All patients having parotidectomy must be warned of the risk of facial nerve damage.

Chapter 40

Neck lumps

A 'lump in the neck' is a common clinical scenario. It is important to have a structured approach to diagnosis and management and to know which neck lumps need urgent referral.

Any of the normal anatomical structures in the neck can become enlarged to cause a 'lump' (Fig. 40.1). In practice most neck masses are derived from the lymph nodes of the neck (cervical adenopathy), the thyroid gland (goitre) or the salivary glands (Chapter 39).

The range of pathologies is very different in adults and children and a different approach is needed.

Lymph nodes

Acute cervical adenopathy

Enlarged tender neck nodes are an expected feature of acute infections in the pharynx or the oral cavity, e.g. acute tonsillitis, infectious mononucleosis. In acute bacterial infection there may be suppuration in the nodes of the neck to form a painful abscess (Fig. 40.2). Treatment is that of the primary condition, e.g. hydration, analgesics and antibiotics as needed.

Persistently enlarged lymph nodes

Children inevitably develop enlarged neck nodes during the course of an upper respiratory infection and as a response to various viral conditions. These enlarged nodes are often multiple and may persist for many months after the infection has subsided. Provided the nodes are of firm uniform consistency, are mobile and

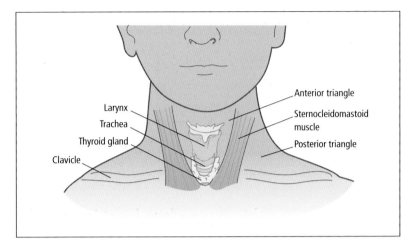

Figure 40.1 The anatomy of the neck showing its division into triangles by the sternoclei-domastoid muscle. The midline structures (larynx, trachea, pharynx, oesophagus and thyroid gland) and the main vessels are in the anterior triangle. The posterior triangle contains nerves, vessels, lymph nodes and muscles.

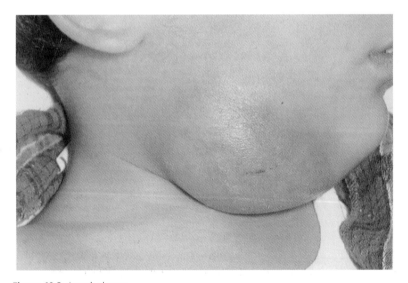

Figure 40.2 A neck abscess.

Box 40.1   Causes of an enlarged neck node

- Acute infection.
- Branchial cyst – a cystic swelling usually in young adults thought to be due to epithelial inclusions in lymph nodes.
- Chronic infection, e.g tuberculosis.
- Lymphoma.
- Malignant disease.
- HIV.
- A variety of chronic inflammatory diseases that cause lymphadenopathy – sometimes called 'pseudolymphoma' and including Rosai Dorfman disease, Kikuchi's disease.

---

non-tender, and have shown no tendency to rapid change or a sudden growth spurt parents can be reassured and the child can be watched.

Indications for referral

- Solitary node (exclude lymphoma).
- Sudden increase in size of nodes.
- Hard rubbery nodes.
- Skin changes in the neck.
- Child generally unwell.
- Severe parental anxiety.
- History suggestive of systemic disease, e.g. HIV infection.

Enlarged neck nodes in **adults** are much more ominous. Head and neck cancer often presents in this way. If there is a clear history of acute infection then treatment with antibiotics is appropriate but a neck node that remains enlarged after 2 weeks needs urgent referral.

Investigations

Most patients with a neck node will now be seen in a rapid access head and neck clinic.

- Endoscopy of the upper aerodigestive tract may reveal a primary cancer.
- Aspiration biopsy cytology (ABC) or fine needle aspiration (FNA) can often confirm a diagnosis at a single clinic visit.
- Ultrasound can help show if a lesion is single or solitary, cystic or solid.
- CT and MRI may be needed to delineate the size of a mass and plan treatment.

Some important causes of an enlarged neck node are shown in Box 40.1.

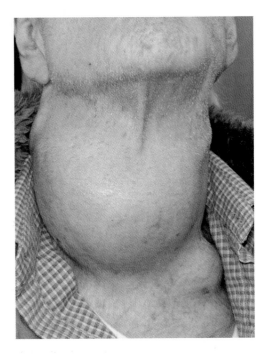

Figure 40.3 Patient with a large goitre. Photo courtesy of Mr SR Jackson FRCS.

Thyroid gland swellings (goitre)

The thyroid gland is situated in the midline of the neck. Two lobes are joined by an isthmus which encircles the trachea (Fig. 40.1). An enlarged thyroid characteristically moves on swallowing (Fig. 40.3). Enlargement can be diffuse, i.e. involving the whole gland or 'nodular'. A nodular goitre may be 'multinodular' or there may be a single focus of swelling in the gland – the more worrying solitary thyroid nodule. The patient may have features of hyperthyroidism, hypothyroidism or more commonly have normal thyroid function ('euthyroid'). Some important causes of thyroid swelling are shown in Box 40.2.

Investigation

A patient with a thyroid swelling should be referred to a head and neck/thyroid clinic. Investigations include thyroid function tests, ultrasound to determine if a nodule is cystic or solid and whether it is single or multiple, and FNA as already described for cervical lymphadenopathy. Technetium scanning (Fig. 40.4) and CT or MRI may be needed.

Box 40.2   Common thyroid swellings

- Cysts.
- Nodules, solitary or multiple, e.g. due to iodine deficiency, reactive hyperplasia.
- Inflammatory, e.g. thyroiditis.
- Benign neoplasms, e.g. adenoma.
- Malignant disease, e.g. carcinoma.

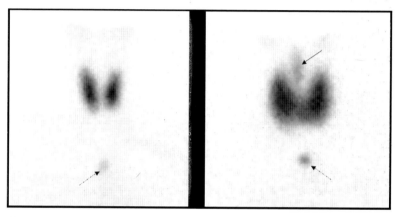

Figure 40.4 Technitium scan showing uptake in the lobes of the thyroid gland. The arrows show a marker at the sternum for orientation and the 'pyramidal lobe' of the thyroid.

Treatment

This will depend on the precise pathology. Not all goitres need treatment. Abnormalities of thyroid gland function may need to be managed with thyroxine or anti-thyroid drugs under the supervision of an endocrinologist. Radioactive iodine under the supervision of a specialist in nuclear medicine is frequently used to destroy overactive thyroid tissue. Most thyroid cancers are associated with a good prognosis if treated early. This will usually require surgery – partial or total thyroidectomy.

Thyroglossal cyst

Goitre is uncommon in children but they not infrequently present with a midline cystic neck swelling (Fig. 40.5) which moves on swallowing and on protrusion of the tongue. This is a cystic remnant of the thyroglossal duct which contributes to the descent of the thyroid gland in the embryo. It may become infected, red and painful. The treatment is surgical excision.

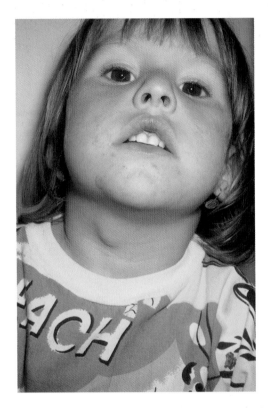

Figure 40.5 Thyroglossal cyst.

Clinical practice point

- An enlarged neck node in an adult is ominous. Refer urgently to a head and neck clinic.

Multiple choice questions

Answer True or False for each question.

1 The external ear:
(a) Is made up of cartilage in the outer third.
(b) Contains part of the facial nerve.
(c) Produces wax.
(d) Contains the 'ossicles' or small bones which transmit sound.
(e) Is lined by glands which produce sticky mucus.

2 When examining the eardrum:
(a) It is best to use the smallest speculum you can.
(b) The light reflex suggests the drum is abnormal.
(c) The normal drum is immobile.
(d) A perforation causes sensorineural deafness.
(e) The pinna should be gently manoeuvred to improve your view.

3 In testing the hearing:
(a) Rinne's test is positive if air conduction is better than bone conduction.
(b) Sensorineural deafness is often corrected by surgery to the middle ear.
(c) Pathology in the inner ear causes conductive deafness.
(d) A unilateral 'dead ear' (i.e. no hearing in one ear) causes profound disability.
(e) Screening the hearing in newborn babies is best done by tuning fork tests.

4 Deafness:
(a) In children is usually profound.
(b) Can be caused by pre-natal infections.
(c) When due to an acoustic neuroma is typically bilateral.

(d) Is a feature of normal ageing.

(e) Is often accompanied by tinnitus.

5   Hearing aids:

(a) Work by amplifying sound.

(b) Need to be worn at all times to be useful.

(c) Batteries can be dangerous in children if ingested.

(d) BAHA (behind the ear hearing aid) requires the insertion of metal screws to the skull.

(e) A cochlear implant stimulates the auditory nerve in children with profound deafness.

6   Conditions of the external ear:

(a) Late treatment of a haematoma of the pinna causes 'cauliflower ear'.

(b) In otitis externa, excessive use of drops causes dermatitis in the ear canal.

(c) Squamous carcinoma of the pinna is mainly a disease of the elderly.

(d) Inert foreign bodies in children need urgent removal.

(e) Microtia in children is often associated with other congenital anomalies.

7   Injury to the eardrum:

(a) A traumatic perforation causes permanent deafness.

(b) Antibiotic drops are needed to prevent infection.

(c) A button battery in the ear canal can cause perforation.

(d) Sensorineural deafness is common after minor head injury.

(e) Requires urgent hospital admission.

8   Otitis media:

(a) Acute otitis media is painless.

(b) Antibiotics are essential for acute otitis media.

(c) In otitis media with effusion the eardrum is perforated.

(d) A cholesteaoma is an accumulation of squamous epithelium in the middle ear.

(e) Sticky mucoid discharge is a feature of chronic otitis media.

9   Acute otitis media:

(a) Is more common in adults.

(b) Is often viral.

(c) Topical antibiotic therapy with eardrops is best in the early stages.

(d) Can be complicated by mastoiditis.

(e) Good analgesia is the mainstay of management.

10 Perforated eardrum:

(a) Can be repaired by myringoplasty.

(b) Causes profound deafness.

(c) Needs no treatment in the presence of a cholesteatoma.

(d) Foetid discharge suggests bony disease.

(e) Is more prevalent in developing countries.

11 Complications of ear infection:

(a) Facial palsy in acute otitis media is usually permanent.

(b) A suddenly protruding ear is a sign of acute mastoiditis in a baby.

(c) Mastoiditis can be safely managed with fluids analgesics and regular clinical review.

(d) In a child with an ear infection, headache may be due to spread to the meninges.

(e) In brain abscess due to ear infection, complete recovery is the norm.

12 Otitis media with effusion (OME)

(a) Is rare in children under 8 years old.

(b) Is more common in children exposed to passive smoking.

(c) Causes imbalance.

(d) Children need grommets in nearly all cases.

(e) Improves following tonsillectomy.

13 Structures that can be involved in referred earache include:

(a) The pharynx.

(b) The larynx.

(c) The perineum.

(d) The temporomandibular joints.

(e) The sternoclavicular joint.

14 Tinnitus:

(a) Is rare in the elderly.

(b) Is often a sign of serious disease.

(c) Can be easily managed by sedation and anxiolytics.

(d) Can be caused by vascular anomalies.

(e) Needs urgent investigation when it is bilateral.

15 Dizziness:

(a) Is often multifactorial in the elderly.

(b) Can be caused by beta-blockers.

(c) In Meniere's disease is typically associated with hemiparesis.

(d) Responds well to vasodilators if caused by peripheral neuropathy.

(e) Benign paroxysmal vertigo is a chronic relapsing condition with a poor prognosis.

16 Bell's palsy:

(a) Is thought to be caused by viral infection in the trigeminal nerve.

(b) Lasts for up to 6 months.

(c) Steroids are contraindicated due to the risk of viral encephalitis.

(d) Some degree of residual paralysis is to be expected.

(e) Is frequently bilateral.

17 When examining the nose:

(a) Crusting and discharge in one nostril in a child is often due to a foreign body.

(b) A good view of the nasal cavity can be had with a disposable torch.

(c) A finding of a deviated nasal septum requires ENT referral.

(d) Rigid endoscopy requires general anaesthesia.

(e) Polyps in children are a common finding.

18 Following nasal trauma:

(a) Complete airway obstruction with a swollen septum is caused by a septal haematoma.

(b) Most fractures need external wiring to get a good result.

(c) It is safe to wait for 7 days before treating a simple facture.

(d) An X-ray of the facial bones is essential to plan treatment of a nasal fracture.

(e) Nasal surgery is an important cause of nasal septal perforation.

19 Nosebleed (epistaxis):

(a) Can be fatal.

(b) Is more likely to be prolonged in the elderly.

(c) May be a sign of coagulopathy.

(d) Packing is well tolerated in children.

(e) Bleeding in children is mostly from the inferior turbinate.

20 Acute sinusitis:

(a) Is commonest in the newborn.

(b) Causes facial pain.

(c) Is usually isolated to one of the paranasal sinuses.

(d) Can give rise to fatal intracranial complications.

(e) Can spread to the orbit.

21 Nasal and nasopharyngeal tumours:
(a) Typically present early due to pain.
(b) Angiofibroma is a disease of adolescent girls.
(c) Metal workers are especially at risk.
(d) Nasopharyngeal cancers are endemic in India and Pakistan.
(e) Curative treatment is mainly with chemotherapy.

22 In 'rhinitis'
(a) Intranasal steroids are contraindicated.
(b) Asthma frequently co-exists.
(c) Nasal polyps are often malignant.
(d) Surgery is the mainstay of treatment.
(e) Allergy to house-dust mite is common.

23 In children with nasal obstruction
(a) Choanal atresia occurs in 1 in 800 births.
(b) Adenoids usually regress by age 4 years.
(c) Snoring is common.
(d) Adenoidectomy is contraindicated in the under 4s.
(e) Bacteria in the adenoids can form a 'biofilm'.

24 Infection in the tonsils ('tonsillitis')
(a) Can be caused by Epstein–Barr virus (infectious mononucleosis).
(b) Complications include retropharyngeal and parapharyngeal abscess.
(c) Staphylococcal infection causes valvular heart disease.
(d) Antibiotics have been shown to greatly improve the speed of recovery.
(e) 'Qunsy' is spread of infection to the neck nodes.

25 Tonsillectomy:
(a) Is almost completely painless with modern techniques.
(b) Is indicated in children with two or more attacks of tonsillitis a year.
(c) Can be complicated by fatal bleeding.
(d) Is helpful in the management of recurrent otitis media.
(e) Should nowadays be reserved for children with immunodeficiency.

26 The larynx:
(a) Laryngeal disease typically presents with hoarseness.
(b) Voice is produced by vibration of the epiglottis.
(c) The vocal cords abduct from the midline to prevent aspiration of fluid into the lungs.

(d) Laryngeal obstruction is quickly fatal unless an alternative airway is established.

(e) Indirect laryngoscopy requires the use of a rigid endoscope.

27 Infections of the larynx:

(a) Can alone cause stridor.

(b) Are more likely to cause airway obstruction in adults than in children.

(c) Respond quickly to steroids.

(d) Are commoner in smokers.

(e) Incidence of *Haemophilus* influenza epiglottitis has increased since the 1980s.

28 Factors predisposing to head and neck cancer include:

(a) Smoking.

(b) Betel-nut chewing.

(c) Exposure to ionizing radiation.

(d) Sedentary occupation.

(e) Bronchial asthma.

29 Cancer of the larynx:

(a) Is commoner in women.

(b) Presents typically with airway obstruction.

(c) Histology is usually adenocarcinoma.

(d) Responds well to chemotherapy.

(e) Prognosis is poor for 'glottic' tumours.

30 Paralysis of one or more vocal cords:

(a) May complicate thyroid surgery.

(b) Can cause aspiration.

(c) Mediastinal lesions usually affect the right vocal cord.

(d) Is a poor prognostic sign in lung cancer.

(e) Treatment does not improve the voice.

31 Airway obstruction in children:

(a) Causes noisy breathing ('stridor').

(b) Inhaled foreign body is commonest in teenagers.

(c) Inhaled peanuts and seeds will usually dissolve without causing any harm.

(d) Large tonsils and adenoids alone are not enough to account for severe obstruction.

(e) Can be relieved by an endotracheal tube.

32 In the pharynx:
(a) An impacted sharp foreign body will usually pass harmlessly into the stomach.
(b) Globus pharynges is commonest in elderly men.
(c) A parapharyngeal abscess can obstruct breathing.
(d) Pharyngeal pouch typically presents in adolescent males.
(e) Untreated carcinoma in the oropharynx is associated with a poor prognosis.

33 Tracheostomy:
(a) Indications include airway obstruction and to facilitate suction.
(b) Incision is best made between the thyroid cartilage and the hyoid bone.
(c) Patients have reduced bronchial secretions for a few weeks after the operation.
(d) Tracheotomy patients are unable to speak.
(e) Long-term risks include stenosis of the airway.

34 Salivary glands:
(a) Mumps causes swelling mainly of the submandibular glands.
(b) Parotid gland stones cause swelling in the floor of the mouth.
(c) Tumours of the submandibular gland involve the facial nerve.
(d) Acute parotitis causes red painful swelling in front of the ear.
(e) Minor salivary glands are found throughout the mouth and tongue.

35 Obstructive sleep apnoea:
(a) Is commoner in women.
(b) When prolonged can affect the cardiovascular system.
(c) Responds to CPAP (continuos positive airway pressure).
(d) Surgery is the first-line treatment for simple snoring.
(e) In children OSA is usually caused by enlarged neck nodes.

36 Neck lumps:
(a) Enlarged neck glands in children need urgent investigation to exclude malignancy.
(b) Squamous carcinoma can be confirmed by cytology of cells aspirated from the neck.
(c) Multinodular goitre is more likely to be cancerous than a solitary thyroid nodule.
(d) Colloid goitre is a premalignant thyroid condition.
(e) Thyroglossal duct cysts are best treated conservatively i.e. left alone.

Answers to multiple choice questions

1 (a) T, (b) F, (c) T, (d) F, (e) F
See Chapter 1

2 (a) F, (b) F, (c) F, (d) F, (e) T
See Chapter 2

3 (a) T, (b) F, (c) F, (d) F, (e) F
See Chapter 3

4 (a) F, (b) T, (c) F, (d) T, (e) T
See Chapter 4

5 (a) T, (b) F, (c) T, (d) T, (e) T
See Chapter 4

6 (a) T, (b) T, (c) T, (d) F, (e) T
See Chapters 5 and 6

7 (a) F, (b) F, (c) T, (d) F, (e) F
See Chapter 7

8 (a) F, (b) F, (c) F, (d) T, (e) T
See Chapters 8–10 and 12

9 (a) F, (b) T, (c) F, (d) T, (e) T
See Chapters 9 and 11

10 (a) T, (b) F, (c) F, (d) T, (e) T
See Chapter 10

11   (a) F, (b) T, (c) F, (d) T, (e) F
     See Chapter 11

12   (a) F, (b) T, (c) T, (d) F, (e) F
     See Chapter 12

13   (a) T, (b) T, (c) F, (d) T, (e) T
     See Chapter 14

14   (a) F, (b) F, (c) F, (d) T, (e) F
     See Chapter 15

15   (a) T, (b) T, (c) F, (d) F, (e) F
     See Chapter 16

16   (a) F, (b) T, (c) F, (d) F, (e) F
     See Chapter 17

17   (a) T, (b) T, (c) F, (d) F, (e) F
     See Chapters 18 and 22

18   (a) T, (b) F, (c) T, (d) F, (e) F
     See Chapter 20

19   (a) T, (b) T, (c) T, (d) F, (e) F
     See Chapter 21

20   (a) F, (b) T, (c) F, (d) T, (e) T
     See Chapter 24

21   (a) F, (b) F, (c) F, (d) F, (e) F
     See Chapter 25

22   (a) F, (b) T, (c) F, (d) F, (e) T
     See Chapter 26

23   (a) F, (b) F, (c) T, (d) F, (e) T
     See Chapters 12, 27 and 28

24   (a) T, (b) T, (c) F, (d) F, (e) F
     See Chapter 29

25   (a) F, (b) F, (c) T, (d) F, (e) F
     See Chapter 29

26   (a) T, (b) F, (c) F, (d) T, (e) F
     See Chapter 31

27 (a) T, (b) F, (c) T, (d) T, (e) F
    See Chapter 33

28 (a) T, (b) T, (c) T, (d) F, (e) F
    See Chapter 34

29 (a) F, (b) F, (c) F, (d) F, (e) F
    See Chapter 34

30 (a) T, (b) T, (c) F, (d) T, (e) F
    See Chapter 35

31 (a) T, (b) F, (c) F, (d) F, (e) T
    See Chapter 36

32 (a) F, (b) F, (c) T, (d) F, (e) T
    See Chapter 37

33 (a) T, (b) F, (c) F, (d) F, (e) T
    See Chapter 38

34 (a) F, (b) F, (c) F, (d) T, (e) T
    See Chapter 39

35 (a) F, (b) T, (c) T, (d) F, (e) F
    See Chapter 30

36 (a) F, (b) T, (c) F, (d) F, (e) F
    See Chapter 40

Index

Note: Page references in *italics* refer to figures